T0100580

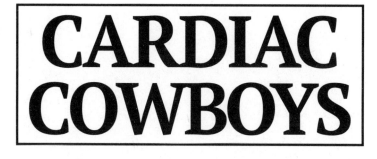

CARDIAC COWBOYS

THE HEROIC INVENTION
OF HEART SURGERY

GERALD IMBER, M.D.

Post Hill
PRESS

A POST HILL PRESS BOOK

ISBN: 979-8-88845-278-3
ISBN (eBook): 979-8-88845-279-0

Cardiac Cowboys:
The Heroic Invention of Heart Surgery
© 2024 by Gerald Imber, M.D.
All Rights Reserved

Cover design by Conroy Accord

Post Hill Press, LLC
New York • Nashville
posthillpress.com

Published in the United States of America
1 2 3 4 5 6 7 8 9 10

For Caroline, Eleanor, and Max,
Thank you for making me smile.

TABLE OF CONTENTS

PREFACE

This book tells the story of the invention of open-heart surgery and the unique people who made it happen. It chronicles the seminal events that took place some seventy years ago and gave rise to the miraculous advances that continue to this day and have brought millions back from the brink of death.

Cardiac Cowboys, by its title alone, should alert the reader that this is meant to be a medical story, not a textbook, nor a hardcore biography. With that said, every fact is well sourced from a wide reading of pertinent volumes that preceded it, an exhaustive search of the medical literature, archival recordings, and in-depth interviews recorded for the production of the podcast of the same name. No suppositions or leaps of faith have been made. This is a high-stakes, true story with all the convolutions of real-life drama. The events happened as reported by reputable sources on the scene. They are neither embellished nor diminished and stand as fact, some absolutely quantifiable, others somewhat subjective and therefore presented as such. The cooperation, competition, courage, and genius of these complex personalities who interacted on the same stage for more than two decades actually invented the lifesaving surgical discipline we take for granted today. No small feat, indeed. The story is so important and so human that embellishment or deviation from fact would be a disservice.

CARDIAC COWBOYS

———●◆●———

The beautiful blonde child wasn't upset when the doctors entered the room. So much of her three years had been spent in hospitals that the white coats and the routines had become simply, routine. The surgeon pulled the buds free from his ears and let the stethoscope dangle from his neck in a casual, practiced gesture. He tousled the child's curls and smiled. He was tall, thin, and ruggedly handsome. A quiet man, his smile radiated sincerity and enough confidence to reassure the parents, barely beyond teenagers themselves, perched nervously on green plastic chairs, holding hands, and waiting for him to speak.

"We're gonna do everything possible. She'll be just fine. You all get some breakfast and wait here. Someone will come by when we finish."

Then he, his senior fellow, and two residents, crossed the hall to a room where a second child with a failing heart slept fitfully beneath the frightened eyes of her parents. The surgeon went through a similar routine, spoke briefly to the parents, left the room, and moved in long strides down the quiet early morning corridor. The young doctors jogged to keep pace as he made his way to the operating suite.

Typically the master of everything around him, from the minute he quietly uttered the words "pump on" to engage the heart-lung machine, he knew things were going south. Tissue tore, sutures didn't hold, and even the best heart surgeon in the world failed to save the child.

The second child seemed to do better. The surgery went perfectly. It was fast and balletic, but in the end they were unable to restart the tiny heart into a sustainable rhythm.

Pulling their masks down from their faces, the senior surgeon and his assistant left the final routines in the cold, still room to their fellows. The young assistant was near tears.

"Is this what it means to be a great heart surgeon? Two dead babies?"

"Tomorrow will be a better day. Tomorrow will be a better day."

INTRODUCTION

In 1948, post war America was booming. The war had finally brought an end to the long Depression and jobs were plentiful. Endless rows of neat little houses were transforming the suburbs. Thousands of shiny new automobiles were rolling off production lines where tanks and fighter planes had been made a few short years before. Food rationing had ended, grocery shelves were well stocked, and butter, eggs, and steaks were back on the table. The cost of living in America had reached an all-time high, and inflation fears troubled Washington. The all-new four door Ford sedan was selling out at a whopping $1,436, and Lucky Strike, America's favorite cigarette, was everywhere, even at the new price of nineteen cents a pack. After years of deprivation, fear, and war, the American dream had come home. The country was at peace, and prosperous.

But the joy was dampened by the fact that its citizens were dying at an alarming rate. Four years of war had taken a dreadful toll of 407,300 young men, but in 1948 alone, more than 500,000 Americans died of heart disease, a staggering annual loss for a nation of 137, 900,000 souls. Heart attacks, caused by what would come to be known as coronary artery occlusion, claimed the overwhelming majority of victims, mostly "healthy" middle-aged men.

At the other end of life, one in every hundred newborns were doomed by congenital heart disease. Too weak to climb stairs, and too fragile to fight off infection, these children invariably failed to thrive and rarely survived the first few years of life.

With little medical insight beyond confirming the cause of death at autopsy, there was nothing to offer beyond a sad prognosis. In both instances, doing nothing was the strategy. The heart was off limits.

Conservative care and unsophisticated medications offered palliation, and some relief...not cure. Not understanding the cause of coronary artery disease made prevention and cure impossible. But this was hardly the case with the stricken children. The frustration of physicians treating children with heart defects was compounded by actually knowing their specific anatomic problems, knowing what would correct them, and being unable to act on that knowledge because the heart was off limits.

But the status quo was about to explode. Change would come from the frigid north, and the steamy gulf coast, not from the elite institutions of the Eastern medical establishment. The result would be a linear, exponential, and complete overhaul of human life expectancy.

This is the story of a small group of surgeons who were the instruments of that change. Individually, each a genius in his own right; ambitious, iconoclastic, flawed, difficult, and in some cases, self-destructive. With the vision and courage that others lacked, they broke the rules, lost lives, and suffered scorn and abuse as they set out on the momentous task of killing the killer.

CHAPTER ONE

HOUSTON, DECEMBER 14, 1964

T he late morning temperature had barely reached fifty degrees, unusually brisk for Houston in late fall. But the oppressive humidity had abated, and the sky was bright and clear when the seventy-year-old Duke of Windsor stepped off the overnight train from New York. The small group of reporters and photographers awaiting his arrival ground out their cigarettes. Notebooks and cameras in hand, they approached respectfully. The Duke appeared rested and fit. Dressed in a severely tailored, double-breasted suit, he wore a thin yellow V-neck sweater and snap-brim fedora against the chill. A slight man, the Duke held himself erect, removed his sunglasses, and smiled to the dazzle of flashbulbs as the cameras captured him and his ever-present wife. The Duchess, dressed in a plaid Chanel suit and long gloves, clung to her husband's right arm, and looked lovingly at him as he faced the cameras.

A highly polished Rolls-Royce limousine in a mini motor-cade delivered the Duke and Duchess to nearby Methodist Hospital, at the Texas Medical Center. In the boardroom of the stark, mid-century modern building, newsreel services and television cameras joined the print reporters for the press conference. In good spirits, the Duke answered questions about his upcoming surgery. Describing his apprehension as no different than one would feel "for even the most minor surgery," he expressed confidence that all would go well, and thanked the reporters for their good wishes.

The following morning, in a sixty-seven-minute operation, an aneurysm the size of a plump orange was removed from the Duke's abdominal aorta and replaced by a simple Dacron tube. Five hours later, he was back in his six-room hospital suite, and according to a hospital spokesman, "smiling, talking, and doing fine." It was all so simple and routine. With typical understatement, the Duke made little of his surgery, but it wasn't every day that a former King of England made his way to Houston, Texas.

In 1964, Houston was an energy hub of barely a million inhabitants, and the home of the NASA manned spacecraft program. It was in no way magnetic enough to attract jaded royalty.

The compelling reason for the pilgrimage was a fifty-six-year-old bespectacled surgeon. Also fairly slight of build, though several inches taller than the diminutive Duke, Michael Ellis DeBakey was in every other way the antithesis of his royal patient. A native of tiny Lake Charles, Louisiana, DeBakey was the son of French Speaking Lebanese Christian parents. Born Dabaghi, the senior DeBakey had changed the family name to the French-sounding version before becoming a successful owner of drugstores, rice farms, and real estate. The family flourished and lived a comfortable, upper middle-class life.

Physically and intellectually, DeBakey was the classic out-sider who had to fight for everything from schoolboy accep-tance to fame and fortune. Skinny, bookish, and unpopular as a child, DeBakey had a dark complexion, heavy eyebrows, and a prominent nose accentuated by oversized, dark-rimmed glasses that seemed part of his face. He neither looked like the other boys in Lake Charles, nor acted like them. He worked at his father's pharmacy, played the saxophone and clarinet, and tin-kered with anything mechanical he could get his hands on. Intense and studious, DeBakey rose above Lake Charles and excelled academically through Tulane University and its med-ical school.

As a young surgeon at Tulane, he outworked and outshone his contemporaries. His interests gravitated to the budding field of vascular surgery, and it would be DeBakey who made it blossom in the public imagination. By the early 1960s, he was the most famous vascular surgeon in a world fascinated by new medical miracles. The procedure upon which the Duke's life depended had been pioneered by others, but was popularized and routinized by DeBakey. The Dacron tube used to replace the weakened wall of the Duke's aorta was the DeBakey graft, a commercial version of one he had fashioned at home on his wife's sewing machine. The surgery performed on the Duke was called a virtuoso performance, and the DeBakey publicity machine made sure the world knew about it.

But the reality was that in 1964, everything about the oper-ation was already quite routine. Everything except the patient and the publicity. The real action was in the heart. Truly *IN the* heart. The story of open-heart surgery had begun a little more than a decade earlier, and though late to the party, DeBakey was about to figure prominently among the imaginative, risk-taking cardiac cowboys who made it happen.

★   ★   ★   ★   ★

The hard-working DeBakey became the first chief of surgery at Baylor Medical College in 1948. Three years later, he made a momentous hire, though he could not yet conceive of the impact it would have on him, Houston, or the world of cardiovascular surgery.

In 1951, the slim, blond, 6'4" Denton Arthur Cooley, twelve years DeBakey's junior, was an adventurous, native Houstonian in a hurry. As an intern at Johns Hopkins, Cooley was a member of the team led by Alfred Blalock that performed the celebrated "Blue Baby" operation that made the public aware of the possibilities of cardiac surgery. It was a bright spot of news in the war-torn world of 1944, and the first hint of the public relations frenzy that would sweep the world twenty-three years later with word of the first heart transplant. Blalock's operation planted a seed in Cooley that would grow into the most prodigious cardiac surgery experience in the world and fuel the most famous feud in medical history.

CHAPTER TWO

1948

G reat scientific advances tend to build gradually on prior work before the tipping point is reached. In the medical sciences, serendipity is not unheard of, but hard work is the rule. The gaping emptiness between recognition and cure of disease is not a vacuum. It is a place of ideas, intense work, and disappointment. Roadblocks, hurdles, goals, and information are shared, and in the background, human competition is the unacknowledged catalyst. Credit and honor are garnered by the lucky few after years of teamwork by the many.

In the world of medicine, great leaps are often made in the living laboratory of war. Under battlefield conditions, even the most conservative physicians throw the rules aside. Desperate situations are met with desperate solutions. Classic examples include the surgical lessons of the Civil War when the seemingly counterintuitive early amputation of gangrenous extremities became a limb-losing, but lifesaving procedure. In that same bloody setting, morphine first came into use on a grand scale to control the pain of the wounded. A medical miracle confirmed on the battlefield, the dark side became obvious as well. While meeting the task of controlling pain, morphine resulted in hundreds of thousands of post-war addicts. Lessons were learned.

In the first World War, more soldiers died of infection than mortal strikes. By World War II, penicillin had changed that, and antibiotics had revolutionized medicine forever. Study after study pushed the needle forward. Lessons learned were chronicled in medical journals, and the methods of study and analysis popularized and expanded the discipline of epidemiology. By applying statistical analysis and scientific method to clinical observation, knowledge was being organized beyond anecdote, triage, trauma, and emergency surgery, and surprising facts began to emerge.

Following the second World War, two unexpected and seemingly unrelated findings struck notes that were impossible for the tone-deaf medical community to ignore. The first was the surprisingly high incidence of coronary artery disease among young American battle casualties. This fact would be driven home still more sharply during the Korean War, when the autopsies of three hundred young men killed in action revealed that 77 percent of these clinically asymptomatic soldiers had significant obstruction of their coronary arteries— the process that proceeds to heart attacks.

The second significant finding took place in Norway, where the Nazi occupation had deprived the population of virtually all meat, fats, and cigarettes. The six years of hardship were accompanied by a dramatic reduction in deaths due to coronary artery disease in a population forced to abstain from smoking and exist on grain, legumes, and vegetables. Immediately after the war, when a "normal" diet and cigarettes were again available, the mortality rate from heart disease sky-rocketed to well beyond pre-occupation levels. These two seemingly random findings sent a signal to the medical community that was impossible to ignore.

At home, where more than five hundred thousand Americans were dying annually from coronary artery disease, nothing was being done about it. This alarming increase in the incidence of heart disease seemed to parallel the return to the good life. Other western countries suffered the same phenomenon, but few on such a grand scale. No other nation lived as richly as America, and heart disease was fast becoming the national plague. The idea that diet and lifestyle were related to atherosclerotic plaque formation blocking the coronary arteries had to be considered. To understand the phenomenon, basic research, clinical studies, sharing of information, and major funding were necessary. The cause had to be identified before the solution could be found.

After nearly two decades of depression and war, the country had become accustomed to grand gestures from government meant to set the path for the future. In war ravaged Britain, the nation rallied behind the National Health Insurance Program. America was not prepared for so radical a departure from the norm, but the health of its people was finally recognized as a critical issue for the most powerful country in the world. Without much resistance, the National Heart Act, a bipartisan bill, was signed into law by President Harry Truman on June 16, 1948. The Act created the National Heart Institute (NHI) within the Public Health Service, and the National Advisory Heart Council. The clearly stated mission of the act was to address and combat heart disease.

Most of the professionals associated with the effort to curb heart disease smoked cigarettes while they brainstormed, drove when they could have walked, and returned home to a big steak dinner, creamy mashed potatoes, and bread and butter—or worse still, margarine—followed by a few more relaxing cigarettes. A well-earned reward for a hard day of improving public health.

★　★　★　★　★

The National Heart Act of 1948 kicked off the beginning of the official fight against heart disease. It was also marked Michael DeBakey's ascension. DeBakey had been Associate Professor of Surgery at Tulane University School of medicine in New Orleans, his alma mater, when the renowned chief of surgery, Alton Ochsner, offered him up for the new position as Chairman of the Department of Surgery of Baylor University College of Medicine. As much as a chair would seem an academic surgeon's dream, it was not an easy step to take. At the time, Baylor was an undistinguished University in Houston. Tulane was the big time, particularly in the South, and particularly in surgery. There, Rudolph Matas and Alton Ochsner, DeBakey's mentors, reigned supreme. Both were internationally respected surgical innovators, and both had seen greatness in the odd-looking, manically-driven young man. As a twenty-three-year-old medical student, DeBakey had developed an ingenious pump for continuous intravenous blood propulsion. The DeBakey pump revolutionized blood transfusions, which at that time were direct person-to-person transfers. The pump accelerated the process, and most critically, didn't destroy fragile red blood cells. Decades later, the DeBakey pump would become an integral part of the first heart-lung bypass machines.

Matas, the elder of DeBakey's two mentors, was considered the father of vascular surgery. He had been a friend, associate, and a patient of William Stewart Halsted, the legendary Johns Hopkins surgeon who had ushered in the era of modern American surgery. Alton Ochsner, who succeeded Matas as Chairman at Tulane, was a pioneering thoracic surgeon of international renown, and proximity to both significant figures greatly influenced DeBakey's career choices.

Lung cancer had not yet been the pervasive ailment it would come to be, but working with Ochsner, DeBakey had noted the high frequency of smokers among the lung cancer patients on their thoracic surgery service. Taking the logical next step, they postulated a link between cigarette smoking and lung cancer. In 1939, the two published a seminal paper on the subject, which was not well received in the tobacco producing South. Ochsner and DeBakey spent years defending their stance to a disbelieving medical community. Through the derision, they held their ground, and their professional bond remained close. Despite the tobacco heresy, Ochsner's position in New Orleans was so exalted that in 1948 he was given the highest civic honor the city could offer, naming him Rex, King of Carnival. DeBakey would have to leave this established fiefdom to become his own master at a medical center, as yet unworthy of the name.

Baylor University College of Medicine had recently relocated from Dallas to Houston. From the rarified vantage point of the ivory tower at Tulane, forty-year-old DeBakey somehow bought into the dream that Baylor could become the Texas Medical Center. But the reality into which he arrived was disheartening. The year before DeBakey's arrival, the medical college had moved from a former Sears, Roebuck & Co. warehouse into a new facility. There were no full-time faculty members, no teaching hospitals, and no surgical laboratories. The Department of Surgery at Baylor was little more than local private practitioners performing routine procedures on private-paying patients and charity cases at the Hermann and Jefferson Davis hospitals.

Several visits to Houston made all of this obvious to DeBakey. What he had initially rejected he began to see as a challenge. Encouraged by Ochsner, he met with Ben Taub, the city's leading philanthropist and chairman of the Jefferson Davis Hospital. Having already made clear his agenda with the dean of the medical college, he was assured by both men of their support for research and teaching beds, as well as a shared vision for the future. DeBakey signed on to what would become a transformative long-term partnership.

Ben Taub and Michael DeBakey were both feverishly driven outsiders who instantly understood and liked one another. Taub, Jewish and unmarried, had devoted his life to building his father's tobacco and candy business into a major regional distributorship from which other successful businesses and a real estate empire had grown. Philanthropy and civic responsibility facilitated Taub's acceptance into Houston society, just as excellence and hard work would pave the way for DeBakey.

With mutual respect and a shared desire to create a great medical center, the two very different men forged a deep friendship. Taub, who often said DeBakey was the only man he had ever known who wasn't interested in money, was one of the very few people with whom DeBakey relaxed. Relaxation for DeBakey meant an hour or two away from work. The two met for coffee on Sunday mornings, after DeBakey's hospital rounds, and as their friendship evolved, they played cards, spoke frequently on the telephone, and shared plans for the medical center they would build together.

Energetic, well-organized, and having done his homework, DeBakey was unfazed by the state of affairs upon his arrival in Houston. From the start, he was unpopular. Ambitious, self-promoting, and openly arrogant about his superior academic credentials, DeBakey made few friends within the medical community. To its practitioners, medicine had always been viewed as a business as well as a profession, and DeBakey, the upstart outsider, used his position to siphon off a good deal of lucrative general surgery from the local surgeons into his own practice. Whatever others thought of him, DeBakey went about his business with single-minded determination. His eighteen-hour work days included skillfully mining money from oil barons in Houston and securing government grants from his contacts in Washington. Very much at the expense of other aspects of life, DeBakey set about building the world famous Texas Medical Center.

★　★　★　★　★

Two years before his arrival, a new Naval Hospital opened its doors on 118 acres of Southeast Houston land. Then, in 1948, President Truman issued an executive order transferring control of the hospital to the Veterans Administration. Already well known in government medical circles from his work during the war, DeBakey was asked to staff the hospital. In short order, he established the Baylor surgical residency and research labs, and the Veterans Administration Hospital became the first hospital fully affiliated with Baylor. Initially, the VA alone funded the expansion and upgrading of the department. It was the first step in making the dream seem like a possibility.

DeBakey enlisted Oscar Creech, a surgeon from Tulane, to become chief of surgery at the VA Hospital. Creech was a well-respected young man on the rise, and it hadn't been an easy sell. But, using his estimable powers of persuasion, as well as common sense, DeBakey added a commodious family home on the park-like hospital grounds as additional incentive. It was a valuable first step, and having a strong ally made the early days that much easier. Creech played a pivotal role in building the surgical residency and establishing research labs. He stayed on for eight years, and in 1956, returned to New Orleans to succeed Alton Ochsner as chief of surgery at Tulane.

DeBakey worked seven days a week. Half-jokingly, he threatened to schedule surgery on Sundays, and complained that the hospital administration insisted on a day off for the OR staff. Vacations and weekends were a waste of time. For DeBakey, work was life. His wife, the former Diana Cooper, had been Chief Surgical Nurse at Charity Hospital in New Orleans, where they met, and at the American Hospital in Paris as well. She knew the drill, and she had seen her husband in action. For the four DeBakey sons, their father was usually absent, so it was Diana DeBakey who attended school plays and baseball games. Church on Sunday mornings fell to her as well, while "Michel," (as Diana called her husband) made his rounds and had Sunday morning coffee chats with Ben Taub. He joined the family later for a big lunch at home, the sole obligatory family time. After Sunday lunch, DeBakey returned to the hospital for a few hours. When his Sunday work was done, he usually stopped by the local Dairy Queen to bring home hamburgers and ice cream for Diana and the boys.

For a family with four active boys, it was hardly a perfect situation. DeBakey woke at five in the morning, breakfasted on Creole style chicory café au lait and a banana, and was off to work by 5:30 a.m. without seeing the children. He often returned home as late as 9:00 p.m. After a few words with the boys and a quick dinner, he worked late into the night behind the closed doors of his study. Sleep was never a priority, and he was fully energized on five hours a night. Meanwhile, the boys were kept busy and well looked after by their mother. DeBakey felt the situation was adequate considering his responsibilities, and his sons were expected to adhere to the strict discipline he imposed on them. But the boys felt cheated, and his absence increasingly irritated Diana.

Meanwhile, relations with the local surgical community were tenuous at best. DeBakey filled the staff with promising young men from outside Houston, despite the fact that this further deepened the divide. At Tulane, he had achieved some renown for special expertise in gastric surgery, for which he had earned a Master of Surgery degree, but his interest had shifted to vascular surgery. Well-grounded in the work of early vascular surgeons like his mentor, Rudolph Matas, DeBakey spent his post residency years of 1935 and 1936 with two pioneering vascular surgeons: René Leriche of Strasbourg, and Martin Kirschner of Heidelberg. At the time, a two-year European tour was considered an important, if expensive, finishing school for surgeons, and DeBakey's trip was financed by his affluent father.

Well trained young innovators like DeBakey were expected to take the next step. Vascular surgery was young, DeBakey was young, and he was prepared to make his mark. Surprisingly, it would be an upstart, and not one of the great professors who made his great leap possible.

★   ★   ★   ★   ★

Early twentieth-century vascular surgery was largely confined to the peripheral vessels, meaning the blood vessels in the extremities, not the life sustaining, major, internal vessels, such as the aorta. Matas developed a successful technique for dealing with weakened peripheral artery walls by using internal sutures to strengthen the ballooned, weakened wall or aneurysm. As the weakened wall of an automobile tire can "blow out" under pressure, so the weakened wall of an artery can "blow out," with disastrous results.

The largest artery in the body, the aorta, is a bit more than an inch in diameter, about the size of a garden hose. Five liters of blood pass through it every minute, under significant pressure. The consequences of a "blow out" of the aorta are obvious and lethal.

While aneurysms of the peripheral vessels are most often due to trauma, aneurysms of the aorta are associated with weakening of the wall, usually due to atherosclerosis. In this process, cholesterol plaques infiltrate the wall of the artery and weaken its structure. Until the mid-twentieth century, syphilitic lesions of the aorta also commonly led to ruptured aneurysms and death. With the advent of penicillin, syphilitic aneurysms became a rarity. Whatever the underlying cause, the surgical objective was to identify the aneurysm and repair it before it burst.

In theory that made sense, but the reality was procedures to contain aneurysms of the aorta were almost universally unsuccessful. Aggressive intervention resulted in massive bloodletting and death. Less invasive procedures were generally ineffective in preventing expansion and rupture of the weakened aorta. Some marginally successful techniques developed in the early twentieth century delayed the inevitable. Still, it was a death sentence.

★   ★   ★   ★   ★

In the fall of 1948, Albert Einstein was found to have an aneurysm of his abdominal aorta. That December, his surgeon wrapped the anterior portion of the aneurysm with Cellophane in the hopes of inducing fibrosis and a thickening of the vessel wall. Odd as the idea of wrapping an artery in commercial packaging might seem, the procedure had gained popularity based on some success. Smaller arteries, mostly in the extremities, had been encircled in Cellophane, resulting in a thickening of the wall and reinforcing the weakness. Feeling it unwise to do the extensive dissection required to free the aorta completely from surrounding tissues to fully encircle it, Einstein's surgeon wrapped only the readily accessible anterior portion with the polymer. The operation was considered a great success.

By bits and pieces, the stage was being set for a dramatic change in aortic aneurysm surgery. DeBakey was poised to be at the center of it, but he wasn't alone. Denton Cooley, after finishing his residency under Alfred Blalock at Johns Hopkins, had spent a year in London with Russell Brock, another pioneering cardiovascular surgeon, and was ready to make his way in Houston, joining DeBakey's staff in 1951.

On his very first day at Baylor, Cooley took off like a rocket. During bedside rounds at Jefferson Davis Hospital, the residents presented a black man with a pulsating mass visible above his clavicle. Diagnosed as an expanding aneurysm of a large vessel coming off of the aorta, DeBakey pushed Cooley for his thoughts. Responding without pause, Cooley proposed to cut it out before it ruptured and repair the aorta. He had done so twice during residency, and the solution seemed obvious. DeBakey sensed impending disaster, but approved the surgery, prepared to bail out the self-confident young surgeon and possibly teach him some humility.

The drama proceeded to the operating room the next morning. To gain access to the aneurysm, Cooley would have to open the patient's chest. The night before surgery, he went to the Veterans Hospital and borrowed a mallet and chisel for the task. In the operating room, he incised the skin with a scalpel, and quickly split the patient's sternum with the mallet and chisel, spread the rib cage open, and went to work. Cooley had clamped and removed the aneurysm and was already suturing the site on the aorta where it had been when DeBakey arrived to watch the operation. Asked for a progress report, Cooley motioned to a stainless steel basin in which the aneurysm had been unceremoniously placed. This seminal moment foretold a great deal about both the future of aortic surgery and the coming relationship between the two men.

An impressed DeBakey was quickly tutored in the procedure, and within a few weeks, four more aneurysm excisions were successfully performed by the two surgeons. At year's end, and to great acclaim, DeBakey presented their four cases, as well as the two Cooley had previously done at Johns Hopkins at a meeting of the Southern Surgical Association.

Earlier in 1951, Charles Dubost, a Parisian surgeon, reported the first successful excision of an actual abdominal aortic aneurysm, replacing the section of aorta with a cadaver graft. This would be analogous to cutting out the weakened, deformed section of the garden hose and inserting another section of hose in its place. Obviously, the water had to be shut off in order for work to move apace. In the case of replacing a weakened section of the aorta, the blood flow had to be clamped off above and below the aneurysm before it was cut out, or, at five liters a minute, the patient would quickly bleed out. The new section (in this case, a specially prepared cadaver aortic homograft of the proper size) would have to be accurately, and quickly, sewn into place before the lack of blood flow damaged vital organs and oxygen deprivation set in. Dubost's procedure worked, and it was a major step forward.

Several months after learning of Dubost's tour de force, DeBakey and Cooley excised an aortic aneurysm and replaced it with a cadaver homograft as well. It was the first time this groundbreaking surgery had been performed in the United States, and the second time in the world. DeBakey referred to the operation as the Dubost procedure, but soon enough, with his publicity machine grinding away, it became DeBakey's operation and was being performed around the country. It was the first time national attention focused on DeBakey, but not yet the leap that launched a legend.

Albert Einstein's cellophane-wrapped aneurysm remained stable for seven years. Then, in 1955, the physicist began suffering severe abdominal pain. On April 14, Einstein was examined at his home in Princeton by Dr. Frank Glenn, chief of surgery at the New York Hospital–Cornell Medical Center, who concluded that Einstein's aortic aneurysm had enlarged and was leaking. He recommended immediate surgery. Time had been on Einstein's side. In the seven years since his original surgery, new techniques had evolved. The aneurysm could now be surgically removed and replaced with either a cadaver graft or the even more recently developed synthetic tubes made of Vinyon-N and Dacron. Glenn had successfully performed several of the cadaver aortic grafts and encouraged the procedure. The seventy-six-year-old Einstein refused, telling Glenn, "I want to go when I want. It is tasteless to prolong life artificially. I have done my share, it is time to go. I will do it elegantly."

Einstein died of a ruptured aortic aneurysm in Princeton Hospital on April 18, 1955.

★　★　★　★　★

In Houston, success followed success. Bumps in the road occurred quietly. Mistakes were made, and patients died as procedures were being fine-tuned. But people with life-threatening aneurysms now had an excellent chance at survival. DeBakey and Cooley reported unheard of volumes of surgical cases, with staggering success. Soon, the mortality risk of aortic surgery in their hands was below 10 percent. Nine out of ten patients who, a few short years ago, would most surely have perished, returned to normal lives. The word was out, and patients flocked to the little medical center in the oil rich port town where DeBakey held court.

Aneurysms can occur in any area of the aorta. While the abdominal aorta has a sizeable section without major branches above the renal arteries, the thoracic aorta, the arching section from the heart to the diaphragm, has several major branches servicing the chest, upper extremities, and the brain. DeBakey and Cooley began performing increasingly complicated surgeries, including removing and replacing the entire, multi-branched arch of the thoracic aorta with a cadaver homograft of similar size. That required the availability of cadaver "tubes" of the same caliber as the artery of the patient. As the operations became more frequent, the availability of properly sized cadaver homografts became increasingly problematic. Obviously, a graft harvested from a five foot, one hundred pound woman would not be a good fit for a six foot, two hundred pound man.

As Houston became a magnet for aneurysm patients, DeBakey grew increasingly aware of the difficulty of matching patient and cadaver grafts. Seeking an artificial substitute for cadaver homografts, DeBakey toyed with the idea of creating a tube from nylon. Unable to find a suitable quantity in the local department stores, he purchased a bolt of Dacron, a malleable new polyester made by DuPont, and became legendary by telling and retelling the story of how he personally fashioned the first Dacron aortic graft on his wife's sewing machine, even reproducing the event for photographers.

In another version of the story, as told by DeBakey's son Michael, his father had never set foot in a Houston department store. But when Michael returned from a trip, DeBakey asked if he had any wash and wear clothes. Michael produced a pair of Brooks Brothers Dacron boxer shorts, which his father then cut up, sewed into a tube, and sent to the dog lab.

His new, Dacron graft was easy to work with, easy to sew, and long lasting. It was perfect for the task and spawned an industry of new materials and weaving techniques from which the vascular surgeon could choose. Soon, commercial grafts for all sections and sizes of the aorta were manufactured to DeBakey's specifications and became generally available. These included the entire thoracic aortic arch, its tributaries, and another world of possibilities was opened for the adventurous surgeon. Synthetic grafts had greater longevity than cadaver grafts, came in a multitude of sizes, and made the procedure markedly easier to perform.

With Cooley at his side, the service grew, and with a steady stream of press releases, the world became aware of Houston's Baylor and the odd-looking, mustachioed, bespectacled man from Lake Charles who was performing miracles. DeBakey thrived on working punishing hours, pushing his team to do more, and making no friends along the way.

Cooley, the handsome, lanky Texan, was present at the inception of all this. In fact, he had taught the master his mastery. He was faster, smoother, and cooler than seasoned surgeons had ever seen. His surgical load was enormous, and he might have dozens of patients in hospital. He worked hard, and quietly, both in the operating room and outside it.

DeBakey, famously explosive in the operating room, and abusive and dismissive to his staff, was generally known to be garrulous, and honey tongued with the outside world. And while DeBakey was making Baylor famous, Cooley was making DeBakey famous. By 1955, routine aortic surgery no longer challenged Cooley, and his thoughts had drifted to the great unknown: open-heart surgery. Meanwhile, the real action in open-heart surgery was taking place up north, in Minneapolis, Minnesota.

CHAPTER THREE

THE RACE TO
CONQUER THE HEART

In the fourth century BC, Hippocrates described, in detail, the symptoms of heart disease. Over the next 2,350 years, the science of observation, diagnosis, and prognosis became increasingly accurate. But the leap from empirical knowledge to action was a leap of courage that few would dare take. As late as the mid-twentieth century, the heart remained strictly off limits. To physically interfere was to invite certain death by bleeding, lethal irregular heartbeat, or no heartbeat at all. This was "fact" supported by myth, anecdotal evidence, and solid scientific, if indirect, experience. Though the heart was no longer believed to be the seat of the soul, the very word "heart" was central to life, and doctors didn't meddle.

In 1881, Theodor Von Billroth, then Europe's most progressive, scientific surgeon, had set the tone in a dictum that would rule for the next sixty years. "Anyone who would attempt to operate on the heart should lose the respect of his colleagues."

By the time America's heart-conscious era began in 1948, it was already clear that the ropelike hardening and obstruction of the coronary arteries was the direct cause of heart attack and adult death, as clearly as congenital abnormalities such as septal defects and abnormal blood vessels were known to doom children. With these facts, made obvious and indelible at autopsy, one would expect the next steps to be obvious as well. Theoretically, they were: close the holes in the hearts of stricken children and restore the compromised blood supply to the heart of adults. Simple. But finding solutions required loosing the bonds of two thousand years of believing the heart was off limits, and finding a way in.

★   ★   ★   ★   ★

Dwight Harken, a thirty-four-year-old chest surgeon assigned to the US Army hospital in London during the second world war, was certainly aware of Von Billroth's admonitions. But faced with a soldier with shrapnel lodged in his heart, Harken's options were clear: do nothing about potential damage of the sharp fragment, or risk taking the patient's life to save it. He chose the latter, stabbed a surgical hole in the heart, blindly inserted a clamp, felt around for the artillery fragment, extracted it, and sewed the heart closed. Harken saved this doomed patient, and then 129 others, without a fatality. With that simple, heroic effort, Harken had quietly opened the floodgates to the heart.

In Philadelphia, surgeon Charles Bailey, was obsessed with the idea of freeing debilitating heart valves frozen by rheumatic fever. The disease was common before the antibiotic age, and its destructive wake persisted for a generation after the acute disease had been controlled. Bailey himself was one of its victims, and his interest was acute. Rheumatic fever often causes the mitral valve between the left atrium and ventricle to become hardened and immobilized by calcium deposits. The flow of blood is impeded, and the heart becomes a very inefficient pump, leading to heart failure. In 1948, Bailey took a chance and stuck his finger into a sick patient's heart. In a blind and bloody moment, he broke open the calcified mitral valve, sutures around his incision tore, and the patient bled to death.

His second patient died as well. The operation was promptly banned at Hahnemann Hospital, his home base. Undeterred, and aware that the knowledge of his mounting mortality figures would put an end to what he was convinced was correct, Bailey stealthily took to operating at different hospitals. He altered techniques and abandoned blunt fracture for a curved knife blade attached to his index finger. Two more patients died. And then they didn't. Bailey's fifth patient went on to live a full life. Soon, enough lives were saved to land Bailey on the cover of *Time*. The gates opened a bit wider, and this time, not as quietly.

In terms of reparative open-heart surgery, the real action, as Denton Cooley realized, was taking place about a thousand miles north of Houston, in Minneapolis. While the great medical centers were dipping toes into these uncharted waters, the unsung staff at the University of Minnesota, a middling medical center, plunged into deep water.

★   ★   ★   ★   ★

In 1948, the population of Minneapolis reached its zenith of 521,718. Electric streetcars were replaced by fume-spewing modern buses, industry was humming, and the city was expanding into new suburbs. The inhabitants of greater Minneapolis and St. Paul were mostly of Scandinavian descent. The punishing winters seemed to be in their blood, and they were there to stay. Homogeneous Minneapolis was known as the most virulently anti-Semitic city in the country, and it certainly wasn't at all welcoming to Black people.

The most prominent local employers were manufacturers, producing grain mills, breweries, and iron mines. Of the businesses surveyed, 63 percent declared they would not hire Jews or Black people. It was an open secret, known to everyone in town, until Eric Sevareid, a young journalist soon to become a national figure, exposed the institutionalized prejudices in a series of scathing articles in the *Minneapolis Journal*. In 1948, more than a decade after Sevareid's exposé, a council on human relations was formed by Hubert H. Humphrey, the thirty-seven-year-old mayor of Minneapolis, but change was slow.

The University of Minnesota toed the line as well. The college remained undistinguished in academic circles, nor was the medical school anything to boast about. Bound by its insularity, students were born, bred, educated, trained, and practiced locally. Here too, the winds of change were slow in coming.

The special ingredient necessary to catalyze change in the medical school was Owen Harding Wangensteen. How Wangensteen felt about the inbred bigotry with which he had lived is less know than his commitment to scientific excellence, which wagged a non-discriminatory tail in his department.

A lifelong Minnesotan, Wangensteen graduated from delivering piglets and inoculating livestock against anthrax at the family farm, to the top of his class at the University of Minnesota Medical School as though it had been preordained. With a prodigious memory, and insatiable curiosity, he became Chief of Surgery at age thirty-one. The youngest university surgery chief in the country, Wangensteen was a man of many ideas. He cemented his reputation that first year by devising a decompressing tube to prevent bowel perforation. The simple, flexible tube inserted through the nose had a weighted tip to help it work its way into the intestine. Once in place, it was connected to a continuous suction device to evacuate air and fluid. The Wangensteen tube proved effective enough to have saved hundreds of thousands of lives. It remains a mainstay of medical practice and put Wangensteen, and the department of surgery at the University of Minnesota, on the map. Wangensteen himself never saw a penny from the worldwide production and use of his invention. He firmly believed that medical progress belonged to humanity, a conviction he instilled in his trainees, which would have enormous repercussions in the future.

After the initial success of his decompressing tube, Wangensteen moved on. Collaborating with physiologist, Maurice Visscher, he structured an academic service around active laboratory investigation. In addition to becoming clinical surgeons, his favored residents were required to earn doctorates in surgery as well. Wangensteen allowed great latitude in their work, followed their progress closely, and was always available for advice. His own work concentrated primarily on gastrointestinal surgery. His longstanding belief in the surgical treatment of ulcer disease was always a sharp point of disagreement with medical colleagues, who believed in diet and medications alone. He was a vocal proponent of the early diagnosis of gastrointestinal cancer, followed by radical surgery. He also believed in the value of a "second look," meaning reoperation some months after initial surgery to determine whether malignancy had recurred.

The generally accepted routine was to avoid additional surgery unless symptoms of recurrence appeared.

Wangensteen published widely, presented papers at surgical meetings, and established the influential "Surgical Forum" at the American College of Surgeons. Though committed to research and teaching, he maintained a vigorous surgical practice, setting modest limits on how much of this earned income he would keep, donating the bulk to the surgical research fund. Often, he refrained from presenting wealthy patients with his bill for services, instead asking them to contribute to the fund what they considered the value of his care.

Fair-haired, with even Nordic features and erect bearing, Wangensteen was a severe-looking, soft-spoken man of principle. Some considered his iron resolve to be simple, hard-headed blindness. Forsaking an opportunity to join a lucrative private practice after his residency, and limiting his income from his academic practice, Wangensteen saw his marriage and family dissolve as he pursued his career. His wife, consumed with material success, was resentful and distant. As his reputation soared and his income remained modest, Helen Wangensteen openly criticized her husband, and began to drink excessively. An already unpleasant marital life was exacerbated by difficult children and child rearing issues. When Wangensteen finally insisted their son be incarcerated in a mental institution after repeatedly running afoul of the law, their marriage, and their family life were over. Helen Wangensteen, chronically depressed and openly alcoholic, had already once attempted suicide. Now, estranged from her other two children as well as her husband, she sued for divorce, and was met with no resistance.

Home pressure relieved, Wangensteen lived not at all unhappily in a single hotel room for several months, and never discussed his situation at work. He met and soon married Sally Davidson, a medical editor, who understood and appreciated his career. Davidson was wealthy in her own right, and finances ceased to be a fraught topic. Wangensteen happily worked long hours, operating, lecturing medical students, teaching resident staff, and overseeing laboratory work.

Wangensteen's teaching sessions were stimulating and exciting and drew many young people into surgery. His lecturing style was simple. He would first outline the big picture and then fill in the fine, interesting details. He knew his subjects thoroughly, always lectured without notes, and engendered an infectious enthusiasm in those around him. His young staff became his family, and their welfare and success were paramount to him. By the time the American Heart Act was passed in 1948, Owen Wangensteen had already recognized the challenge and geared up his staff to meet it. Although he had little personal interest in performing open-heart surgery, Wangensteen began assigning research projects involving the physiology of the heart and encouraging animal experimentation to familiarize the young surgeons with the surgical anatomy he was certain they would soon need to know.

Early open-heart surgery was often a violent, impulsive business, such as Bailey fracturing a calcified valve with a finger, or Harkin removing shrapnel from the heart. These were procedures done blindly in a pool of blood, but they proved beyond a doubt that the heart was not at all off limits. Still, no significant surgery had been attempted within the heart for two simple reasons. First, the beating heart, spewing blood at five liters a minute, would require incalculable transfusion for even the most direct procedure. Second, a corollary of the first, was that to interrupt the pumping action either by stilling the heart, or clamping off the major vessels from it, would result in oxygen deprivation of the brain. Just over four minutes without oxygen could be sustained without permanent brain damage. A very small window indeed.

Understanding the limitations this implied on heart surgery, Wangensteen assigned Clarence Dennis, one of his bright, young Minnesota men, to the task of building a machine that could take over blood pumping and oxygenating functions, effectively bypassing the heart. A heart-lung bypass machine. It was an important idea, but it did not originate with Wangensteen. For reasons not initially related to open-heart surgery, one man, John Gibbon, had been devoted to the idea of a heart-lung bypass machine since 1931. It was a teasing bit of science fiction that seemed as if it should be within reach, but time and again, it wasn't. Others who had dabbled with rudimentary organ perfusion devices included aviator Charles Lindbergh, and Nobel Prize winner Alexis Carrel, at the Rockefeller Institute. Both national heroes, Lindbergh and Carrel did interesting seminal work, but fell from public grace for their shared Nazi sympathies.

Wangensteen recognized the absolute necessity of bypassing the heart and lungs for the full potential of heart surgery to be realized. And in his quiet way, he cast his lot in that pursuit. The newly born cardiac surgery division in Minnesota was Owen Wangensteen's favored child, and he hoped to have that child on the road to winning the Nobel Prize.

CHAPTER FOUR

BEGINNING

The adult human heart is roughly the size of a clenched fist. It weighs three hundred grams—about two thirds of a pound—and is almost entirely muscle. Within this fist of muscle are four chambers: two reservoir-like upper chambers—the atria—and two muscular lower pumping chambers—the ventricles.

Each day, the heart beats about one hundred thousand times and pumps two thousand gallons of blood. It is the functional center of the cardiovascular system. In the simplest terms, it's a pump. But it's a pump with a very complex electrical system that exquisitely times its operation and coordinates its output with the needs of the body.

The cardiovascular system, the accepted medical term, interchangeably called the circulatory system, refers to the network of veins, arteries, lungs, and heart that collect, oxygenate, circulate, and recirculate blood. Since it is truly a closed system, one can begin observing the process from any point. A logical place to start is the collection of oxygen depleted, carbon dioxide rich blood by the small capillaries and veins throughout the body. These little vessels from the various organs connect to increasingly larger veins, and ultimately deliver blood to the right atrium of the heart through two great veins, the upper, or superior vena cava, and the lower, or inferior vena cava.

The right atrium acts as a reservoir for the deoxygenated blood and allows it to enter the right ventricle beneath it through the tricuspid valve. The right ventricle then contracts and propels the dark-colored, deoxygenated blood across the pulmonary valve into the pulmonary artery, which delivers it to the lungs. The valves allow the propulsion of blood without permitting backflow into the various chambers.

In the lungs, carbon dioxide is released, and life-giving oxygen is replenished and carried in the hemoglobin of the red blood cells. The freshly oxygenated, bright-red blood from the lungs is returned to the heart via the pulmonary vein, where it collects briefly in the left atrium, and passes down through the mitral valve into the muscular left ventricle. The muscular left ventricle then pumps the blood out through the aortic valve into the aorta. From the aorta, blood flows into the distributing arteries, which supply oxygenated blood to the muscles and internal organs, including the brain, via the carotid arteries. The coronary arteries nourish the oxygen-hungry, constantly-working heart muscle itself.

In this continuous cycle of life, oxygenated blood must reach every organ of the body, but two specific areas are of immediate concern, the oxygen-demanding brain and the heart muscle itself, which rapidly succumbs to oxygen deprivation by death of muscle or myocardial infarction: heart attack.

★ ★ ★ ★ ★

Central to this elegant circulatory system, the heart can beat some four billion times, sustaining life for a century. When all is functioning properly, the system needs no maintenance. Ultimately, however, there are glitches in every system, and the cardiovascular system is not an exception. Numerous medical options are available to deal with a multitude of possible situations, but when surgical repair of the heart is attempted, it can take two forms. The first form of true heart surgery takes place with the heart beating and blood circulating. Operating inside the heart with blood rushing at a gallon a minute is a nightmare. Visibility is nearly impossible, and in addition to the danger of mistakes made operating blindly, there is the all-too-real risk of rapid, lethal blood loss. Nevertheless, a number of early procedures were performed under these circumstances. Speed, dexterity, and the relative simplicity of the tasks defined the work. This is where heart surgery began.

Most heart surgery is performed with the heartbeat stopped, which makes the whole process easier to visualize and perform. There have been exceptions, early and late, but generally, that's the rule. The heart can simply stop beating because of surgical intervention, hypothermia, or intentionally through the use of drugs. The obvious issue in dealing with the still heart is the ability to restart the heartbeat in a regular rhythm at the completion of surgery.

But when the pumping heart is stopped, vital organs are immediately deprived of oxygenated blood. Sustained oxygen deprivation leads to organ shutdown, beginning with brain damage and heart muscle loss. Therefore, if the beating heart is to be stopped to facilitate surgery, an alternative method of providing oxygenated blood is required to support life.

If circulation could be diverted to exclude the heart and lungs using a pump other than the heart, and an oxygenator other than the lungs, the surgical field would be virtually bloodless, oxygenated blood would nourish vital organs, and the possibilities for heart surgery would be limited only by the ingenuity and skill of the surgeon. All that was required was a substitute for the heart and lungs. Conceptually simple, but functionally challenging.

That search had begun years earlier, and not at all with open-heart surgery in mind.

★　★　★　★　★

In 1931, John Heysham Gibbon, Jr. was a research fellow at the Massachusetts General Hospital, under the distinguished Professor Edward Churchill, a surgical leader of the time. One of Churchill's patients, a fifty-three-year-old woman, was to have been discharged from the hospital following uneventful gall bladder surgery. One afternoon, she was biding her time comfortably in the solarium when she suddenly cried out in pain and fell forward from her wheelchair. Churchill, on examining his patient, diagnosed massive pulmonary emboli, essentially, blood clots in the lungs. She was rushed to the operating theater where Gibbon was assigned a bedside vigil with orders to call Churchill if the woman's condition worsened. Ultimately, her vital signs weakened, Gibbon alerted his chief, and Churchill rushed to the operating room and slashed opened the moribund woman's chest. Massive blood loss accompanied an unsuccessful attempt to remove the clots from her lungs and the patient died.

Young John Gibbon was stricken, standing by helplessly as he watched the woman die. Unable to dispel the feeling of uselessness, Gibbon mused to himself, and ultimately to Churchill, that if they could somehow have bypassed her pumping heart, the clots could have been removed in an organized fashion, and she could have been saved. Churchill recognized the enormity of the task and the unlikelihood of success, but impressed by the young man's enthusiasm, he encouraged Gibbon to take his idea to the lab.

Gibbon and his wife Mary, his assistant from nearly the beginning of his quest, spent long hours over many years in the animal laboratory working on constructing rudimentary bypass machines, and making slow but steady progress. By 1937, then at the University of Pennsylvania, Gibbon reported having kept a cat alive for four hours on his heart-lung bypass machine. When the war intervened, his work was put on hold. Upon returning from the China Burma theater of war, Lt. Colonel Gibbon followed his obsession to Jefferson Medical College in Philadelphia, where he would later become Chief of Surgery. Shortly after returning, he was introduced to Thomas Watson, the CEO of IBM. Fascinated with the idea, Watson offered financing and a team of engineers to help in the development of a machine applicable to humans. With the improved technology, Gibbon was able to keep laboratory dogs alive for more than an hour. Dogs are more complex animals, and more comparable to humans in their physiological reactions than cats. Soon, the stage was set for a human trial, and Gibbon was now thinking of attempting open-heart surgery. He had been communicating and sharing ideas and plans with Minnesotan

Clarence Dennis since the late 1940s. By the early 1950s, both had nearly a 100 percent success rate bypassing and reviving dogs, and both were edging toward the first human use of the heart-lung bypass machine.

★　★　★　★　★

In Minnesota, on April 6, 1951, With Wangensteen's active encouragement and gentle pushing, Dennis brought his machine to the operating room. The patient he chose for the first human bypass operation was Patty Anderson, a six-year-old with severe cardiac symptoms and a loud murmur indicating an atrial septal defect, a hole in the wall between the atria and the upper collecting chambers of the heart. Patty had been chronically short of breath, easily fatigued, and plagued by pneumonia. With little in the way of diagnostic tools, it had been impossible to pinpoint the exact location of the lesion.

During surgery, the preoperative diagnosis was found to be incorrect, and Dennis faced a far more profound defect, which he could not successfully correct. Patty Anderson died on the operating table, but the bypass machine had performed perfectly for forty minutes. In the period before surgery, it was Richard Varco, the first assistant on Dennis's team, who had developed a close relationship with the parents, and it was he who Dennis delegated to deliver the devastating news.

Dennis remained stoic and undeterred, and a few days later, with every technical reason to be optimistic about his bypass machine, he operated on two-year-old Cheryl Judge. She, too, had been diagnosed with an atrial septal defect. This time, the diagnosis was correct. Tragically, one of the technicians operating Dennis's immensely complicated machine blundered, and the child died purely from technical error. Air had been inadvertently pumped into her circulatory system, resulting in a lethal air embolism. C. Walton Lillehei, a junior member of the surgical staff at Minnesota, was in the operating room as one of several assistants. Lillehei, whose lab adjoined Dennis's, had great respect for the senior surgeon, but misgivings about the complicated apparatus that required sixteen people to operate. Given the chance, it would not be the way he would approach the same problem.

Shortly after the two surgical deaths, Dennis left Minnesota to become Chief of Surgery at the State University of New York Downstate Medical Center in Brooklyn. Part of his contract required Downstate to purchase his lab equipment and his bypass machine. Dennis quietly moved forward with his work, but he had missed the window of primacy. Having failed the opportunity to be first, Dennis became just one of the many, always helping others, always making surgical progress, and not at all distressed that fame and fortune had eluded him. Dennis, among very few other unrecognized pioneers, would stand apart from the ambitious competition that followed him into the newsreels.

In February of 1952, ten months after Dennis's attempts, Gibbon brought his own heart-lung machine into the operating room. He was ready. He had seen the future and had conceived and built the first operational heart-lung bypass machine. He had worked diligently, quietly, and confidently. Whomever followed, and to whomever success came first, it was his concept and his invention, and he truly believed a Nobel was within his grasp. But in his attempt, he too lost his first bypass patient, again, due to misdiagnosis beyond his surgical abilities, as had Dennis.

With the modalities available today, such blatant diagnostic errors are a rarity. The heart can be visualized and measured in all its aspects and functionality. This had not been the case in 1952. Despite the discovery of cardiac catheterization in 1929, it had been virtually ignored, and its use as a diagnostic tool was still in its infancy. By the late 1940s, it had progressed to the point that by sampling the oxygen content of blood obtained through catheters threaded into the chambers of the heart, one could diagnose a ventricular septal defect by the high oxygen content of blood in the right ventricle, which normally contained deoxygenated blood about to be pumped to the lungs. With the hole in the wall between the ventricles, the high pressure left ventricle forced oxygenated blood into the deoxygenated pool in the right ventricle. Similarly, the finding of oxygenated blood in the right atrium would suggest a hole in the wall between the right and left atria, an atrial septal defect. But the actual pathological anatomy was often not as simple and clear cut as the blood samples would indicate.

Each congenital defect in the heart causes a particular sound accompanying every heartbeat. These abnormal sounds, called murmurs, reflect the irregular blood flow through a defect like a hole in the septum, or through an abnormal valve. Over the years, following medical histories and ultimately autopsy findings taught physicians to associate the murmurs transmitted through their stethoscopes with the heart defects that caused them.

The information from the rudimentary catheterization and the nature of the murmur were often all the cardiologists had to go on. They were often incorrect, and often misled the surgeons with tragic results.

Since diagnosis was still an inexact science, and children often had both atrial septal defects and ventricular septal defects, as well as complex combinations including other malformations, it was impossible to distinguish the problem authoritatively. Children with one, both, or combined defects, all presented with pronounced murmurs, heart failure, difficulty breathing, and failure to thrive normally. They were often pathetically skinny and easily fatigued, but as a rule, not unhappy with their lot. They knew no other life. They were repeatedly hospitalized with pneumonia and were blissfully unaware that mortality could come before their next birthday. Parents came to believe what cardiologists and pediatricians knew: the child would die without intervention. The problem was that intervention had so far resulted only in prematurely dead children.

★   ★   ★   ★   ★

Surgical specialization in the mid-twentieth century looked nothing like it does today. Although the American Board of Surgery was founded in 1937, the bulk of surgery in the country was still being performed by general practitioners. Specialized residencies and certification had already taken root, but medical licenses allowed the licensee then (as now) to practice both medicine and surgery. This was a stance supported by the AMA at the time, for reasons both good and bad. The good reason was that it brought medical care close to home, where it was needed. There were far fewer specialists, and access to them was often limited in all but affluent urban areas. The bad reason was that surgery was both lucrative and interesting. Family doctors believed that for most surgeries they were as able as fully trained specialists. Some might have been. Most were far from it. But it was the family doctors, not the specialists, who controlled the American Medical Association. Surgical societies and surgical meetings began to flourish after the war. They too were less specialized, and generally included most branches of surgery. General surgeons, for instance, were still doing orthopedic surgery as well. And neurosurgery had only recently slipped from the grasp of the general surgeon.

In the absence of any dedicated cardiovascular surgeons, most of the advances edging toward open-heart surgery were presented at surgical association meetings. The audiences were comprised of general surgeons, and often what were considered great breakthroughs for the few were, at most, interesting oddities for the many.

In April of 1950, the American Surgical Association met in Colorado Springs, Colorado. There, Wilfred Bigelow, a Canadian surgeon, presented an impressive paper on the use of hypothermia (cooling of the body) to reduce metabolism. His plan was to adapt the technique to open-heart surgery. Conceptually, instead of the human brain tolerating four minutes of anoxia, the time might easily be doubled by slowing metabolic needs. Operating on dogs, Bigelow cut off circulation for twenty minutes, then re-warmed the dogs with no obvious ill effects. But dogs are not humans, and the next leap would be a risky one.

The adventurous Charles Bailey was in the audience. Bailey saw the possibilities and wasted little time taking the concept to the operating room. Soon after the meeting, he attempted using hypothermia to allow the brain to tolerate a few more minutes without oxygen. This, he postulated, would give him enough time to correct an atrial septal defect. Bailey was first to the hypothermia party, but his attempt failed when the patient, an adult woman, sustained a lethal air embolism, the result of air bubbles in the circulatory system, the same issue that had led to the death of Dennis' second patient. This time, it occurred without a heart-lung machine and operator error. The lesson learned: a heart opened surgically harbors ambient air, which must be evacuated and flushed from the system. Another tragic bump to be smoothed out on the road to progress.

CHAPTER FIVE

LEWIS AND LILLEHEI

D espite Bailey's setback in Philadelphia, the idea of hypothermia had obvious merit, and others would follow the
thread. After the departure of Clarence Dennis. Wangensteen
reached into his bullpen for two men uniquely suited to enter
the fray. John Lewis and Walt Lillehei, newly graduated from
residency training, had assisted Dennis in the lab and in surgery
and were up to date on the latest techniques. Both were present
in Colorado Springs for Bigelow's hypothermia lecture, were
excited about the prospects, and began related experiments as
soon as they returned to Minnesota.

Lewis and Lillehei were great friends. Native Minnesotans
who roomed together at medical school, they had been in the
army together, and did their surgical residencies and advanced
degrees in surgery together. From his arrival in the department, Lillehei was the chief's favorite, and it was he who
Wangensteen had named to head cardiovascular surgery, whatever that meant at the time. But Lillehei had recently under-
gone extensive surgery at Wangensteen's hand for cancer of

the parotid gland and had lost four months to the surgery and recovery. By default, Lewis had become senior among the new staff surgeons. Wangensteen, respecting the hierarchy, chose Lewis to move the hypothermia project from the dog lab to the operating room.

Animal experimentation itself has always had organized, zealous opposition, and often for good reason. Legions of animal experiments have crossed the imaginary line of brutality in the name of science. Over the years, a tenuous détente was reached, and more humane guidelines were established. Besides defending the practices, one has to believe in the value of the experiment, and the hope that successes with laboratory animals were somehow transferrable, or beneficial, to humans, and not simply tinker at the cost of animal lives. The argument was that saving human lives takes precedence. It was a strong argument, but the ethical questions don't stop there. New surgical techniques typically face safety and morality issues, as well as restrictions of social mores. Animal experimentation was the least contentious issue when human lives were clearly at stake.

As the era of open-heart surgery began, it appeared that lifesaving repair of many congenital defects was very likely possible. The problem was doing it safely. Experimental solutions for diseases of the coronary arteries, heart valves, and potentially lethal heart rhythms were still beyond the horizon. But, theoretically, congenital defects such as atrial and ventricular septal defects should be repairable. See them, sew them, and save a life.

In the absence of other simple cause and effect situations, the early work in open-heart surgery was directed at methods to salvage these otherwise doomed children. The defects lent themselves to simple correction once the surgeon was in the heart. But there was the haunting ethical conundrum. Was it really acceptable to try an experimental procedure on a child with a slim chance to grow to adulthood with the looming possibility of an even earlier demise in the pursuit of an unproven cure? Facing these decisions made most surgeons tread very carefully, if at all. Mistakes made in the laboratory were considered part of the learning curve, necessary to minimize risk before new procedures were brought to the operating room. Once in the operating room, the lives of children were on both sides of the equation.

Hypothermia was a proven physiological phenomenon. Lowering metabolism definitely forestalled tissue damage, and it seemed a natural first step. That was solid ground. Using it to buy time for open-heart surgery was a new application, but not a new concept. Using ice baths and a refrigerating unit to reduce a child's body temperature below thirty degrees centigrade, while probably safe, was unknown territory. For that matter, so was the process of rapid rewarming to follow. Of course, the ultimate surgeon's nightmare was misdiagnosis, or surgical failure. For some, taking these risks, real as they might be, seemed appropriate weighed against a shortened lifespan, if not imminent death of a child.

John Lewis's first patient was a five-year-old girl named Jacqueline Johnson. She was small and weak, but in little danger of immediate death. According to the pediatric cardiologists at the Variety Club Heart Hospital at the University, her future was bleak without surgical intervention. The preoperative diagnosis had been atrial septal defect, and Lewis believed that with a bloodless field, he could get in, sew the defect closed, and restore circulation in fewer than five minutes. How much leeway hypothermia actually afforded humans before loss of brain cells remained unknown. That was the real experiment. Five minutes seemed safe.

On September 2, 1952, in the operating room at University Hospital, Jacqueline Johnson was anesthetized and wrapped in a cooling blanket, with a thermometer inserted into her rectum. Over the course of more than two hours, her temperature was monitored, and gradually lowered to 28 degrees centigrade. Lewis feared that lowering it further, as Bigelow had in laboratory animals, ran the risk of causing ventricular fibrillation, a lethal heart rhythm. As cooling progressed, Jacqueline's heart rate slowed, and respirations all but ceased. Lewis prepared to make the incision.

Richard Varco, as first assistant, stood across the table from Lewis. This was unusual in the surgical hierarchy. Varco was a far more experienced surgeon than Lewis and senior men rarely serve as assistants to their juniors, except in teaching situations. The arrangement spoke to the momentous task Lewis was about to undertake. As second assistant, Lillehei stood to Lewis's right. After a moment of silence, John Lewis drew his scalpel in a horizontal direction across the mid-right chest, toward himself. The muscles between the ribs were cut, and the small bleeding vessels secured in hemostats. Fine silk sutures were tied around the tips of the clamps, the chest entered, and the ribs spread apart. Lillehei and Varco held retractors specifically placed by Lewis to allow him maximal visibility. The major blood vessels coming to and from the heart were identified and gently encircled with wide tapes to halt blood flow and prevent catastrophic injury to them. Lewis then entered the tiny heart through an incision in the wall of the right atrium. After the blood within the heart was suctioned off by Varco, Lewis was presented with a clear, virtually bloodless field. He was immediately able to identify the predicted atrial septal defect in the middle of the field, well within reach, and he easily sewed it closed with silk sutures. While others glanced at the clock, Lewis focused. Five and a half minutes had passed without blood flow to the brain by the time the entry wound to the heart had been closed and the ties on the great vessels released. But there was no heartbeat.

Lewis began manual massage of the tiny heart between his fingers. Then, after a moment of hesitation, Jacqueline Johnson's heart contracted spontaneously, and resumed beating in a normal rhythm.

After thirty-five minutes of rewarming in a farm trough filled with hot water, her rectal temperature rose to a low normal 36 degrees centigrade. Jacqueline was returned to her room. She had an uneventful recovery and was discharged from the hospital eleven days later. The world's first survivor of open-heart surgery.

For a brief period, Lewis became an international celebrity. Square jawed and handsome, with a full head of curls and a ready wit, Lewis was perfect for the role. He was thirty-six years old.

Hot on his heels was Henry Swan, chief of surgery at the University of Colorado, who had practiced hypothermia on three hundred dogs before attempting human surgery. Swan was incensed that young Lewis had operated on only thir-ty-nine laboratory dogs and had the reckless audacity to take the procedure to the operating room. Swan considered himself the leader and there had been others in the running. Charles Bailey had made his first attempt at open-heart surgery under hypothermia a month before Lewis and failed. Bailey suc-ceeded on his next try, but success came a month after Lewis's, and he wasn't first. Wilfred Bigelow, who had proposed the idea of open-heart surgery under hypothermia, could not find a willing surgical candidate in Toronto, and missed the opportunity that should have been his.

Swan openly resented both Lewis's success and Lewis himself. In one instance, he publicly congratulated Varco on the operation and refused to mention Lewis, the operating surgeon. As a department chief, and an older, respected surgeon, Swan did everything in his power to take the spotlight from Lewis. In this, he largely failed as Lewis basked in months of international accolades for his success.

The thorny issue of laboratory preparation and surgical firsts is a story that would play out repeatedly in the world of heart surgery and dust up a far greater international storm in the race to transplantation. Fourteen years later, Norman Shumway, the leader in heart transplant research, who all expected to perform the first human heart transplant, would say, "no one remembers the second man to reach the North Pole."

★ ★ ★ ★ ★

Lillehei was a man who did not know jealousy. He was both genuinely happy for Lewis's success, and immediately aware that the time constraints of hypothermia would make more complicated open-heart surgery impossible. As friends, Lewis and Lillehei were as unusual a pair as one could envision. Lillehei was as devoted to Lewis as he would ever be to any friend. He respected and cared for him both for their shared past and for Lewis's care and friendship during Lillehei's recovery from surgery. But they were cut from different cloth. While Lillehei was taciturn, quiet, and respectful at work, Lewis was given to speaking his mind in all circumstances. No one was spared his sharp barbs, including the chief, Owen Wangensteen. He was amusing, intellectual, and an extremely gifted surgeon. Lillehei, on the other hand, had been an administrator in the army, spent half of his residency in research, and had little experience in clinical surgery when he graduated to the senior staff level. But he was a quick study. He watched, learned quickly, and was an unusually imaginative surgical thinker, totally obsessed by the problem at hand. He would listen, think, decide, and move directly forward with the tonnage of a great vessel. Lillehei's off mode was drinking and partying. Lewis's was writing, painting, and music.

In Philadelphia, John Gibbon had already failed in his first human use of his heart-lung machine seven months before Lewis's successful atrial septal defect (ASD) repair under hypothermia. Version two of the machine worked perfectly. Developed with the aid of up-to-date IBM technology, it was based on a large screen oxygenator over which blood was propelled by pumps devised twenty-one years earlier by Michael DeBakey. At surgery, the machine allowed adequate time to correct a misdiagnosed defect beyond the ability of the surgeon to correct. Gibbon was ready to try again.

On May 6, 1953, eight months after Lewis performed the first successful open-heart surgery, Gibbon operated on an eighteen-year-old young woman with an ASD, again using his heart-lung machine. With twenty-six minutes on complete bypass, he corrected the defect and a healthy patient left the hospital, the first patient surviving surgery on a heart-lung machine. This had been a breakthrough of great importance, and a point of differentiation that would play a pivotal role in the rapid ascent of open-heart surgery. But it received very little attention at the time.

Gibbon, a reserved, Princeton-educated, fifth-generation physician, was as quiet about his success as he was about his prior failure. He also harshly judged any method other than the bypass machine. Very much unlike his contemporaries, Gibbon had been described by Denton Cooley as, "a surgeon who wanted to be a poet....He sought no publicity, and was modest to a fault."

Most cardiovascular surgeons learned of the first successful use of the heart-lung bypass machine by reading about it in the ubiquitous *Time* magazine, a week after the fact. There were no press conferences, and no announcements. The first time Gibbon spoke publicly about his cases was the following fall, at a conference organized by Wangensteen in Minnesota. Afterward, the speech was published in *Minnesota Medicine*. It had never been published in a major, peer reviewed, medical journal.

With self-effacing good manners, Gibbon allowed himself to be defined by his work, and freely shared the fruits of his years in the lab. Even after his partnership with IBM ended, Gibbon's machine was the most advanced among the few bypass machines being actively developed. He had shared knowledge with Clarence Dennis, knowing that Dennis might make an earlier attempt to employ a version of his own bypass machine and would share it again with another colleague.

Following quickly on his great success, Gibbon operated on two children, but both died on the table. Devastated, John Gibbon, the inventor of the heart-lung bypass machine, never again performed open-heart surgery. He declared a moratorium on both the use of his machine, and on all cardiac surgery at Jefferson. By the time he considered it safe to resume, he had named a junior as his successor.

Gibbon remained professor and chairman of surgery at Jefferson Medical College, performed other surgical procedures, and regularly attended cardio thoracic surgery meetings. He achieved his goal of developing a bypass machine and had withdrawn permanently from open-heart surgery.

Gibbon was awarded the prestigious 1968 Albert Lasker Award for Clinical Medical Research, and although his name had been put forward for the Nobel Prize he sought, it had eluded him.

CHAPTER SIX

THE NEXT STEP

Following his breakthrough in September of 1952, Lewis continued operating with considerable success. For most of the year, he was the only surgeon in the country regularly performing open-heart surgery. He repaired sixty atrial septal defects under hypothermia, with a median circulatory occlusion time of four minutes and forty-five seconds. Pushing the envelope, he had a patient survive seven minutes and forty-five seconds of anoxia. Lewis's fame grew, and his patients came to include adults as well as infants. Hypothermia as a modality for open-heart surgery was at once both excellent and limiting. For a short window, F. John Lewis *was* open-heart surgery, but it was a star that was soon to fade.

As Lewis basked in his success, Lillehei was consumed by the idea of expanding the reach of heart surgery. He continued working as a general surgeon, while supervising his assistants in the laboratory. His full-time lead researcher, Morley Cohen had, with Herbert Warden, another resident, begun working on something called the azygos factor. The concept was that the azygos vein above the heart delivered some 10 percent of circulating blood back to the heart even after major vessels are clamped off. Experiments in the dog lab had proven this blood flow was enough to sustain brain function for twenty minutes while the heart was isolated. Cohen measured the flow carefully by collecting the blood in a condom before returning it to circulation. It was knowledge they would use to calculate just how little oxygenated blood was enough.

As successful as it was in the dog lab, the evidence of azygos perfusion was not well-received when presented for human implementation. A number of other early innovative attempts briefly made it into the operating room, including a technique devised by the important, and particularly self-important, two-time Lasker award–winning Harvard surgeon, Robert Gross. His technique involved a funnel continuously delivering oxygenated blood into the heart, and essentially. working blindly in a sea of blood.

Commenting on Gross's presentation at a meeting, Lillehei, direct as ever, rose and made the point that being able to see when one operates is better than operating blindly. It was a simple and proper observation, delivered flatly, and without softening preamble. Thus, making a powerful, lifelong, enemy. The comment was typical of Lillehei, who spoke frankly, never politically, and never intending his blunt remarks to be hurtful. Nor did he take offense at others poking holes in his own pet project of the moment. Lillehei seemed to function insulated from many of the courtesies generally observed by others. It was an aspect of his personality that oddly contrasted with his easy likeability and pleasant demeanor.

One Friday afternoon, during Lillehei, Warden, and Cohen's weekly research meeting at the Parker House, their favorite spot for martinis and music, Cohen told Lillehei that his wife was pregnant. After congratulations and toasts, Warden remarked that he and Cohen had been discussing how the placenta bypassed the not yet functional lungs of the embryo, and using someone else's circulation, would be a great way to sustain life during surgery. Lillehei fell still, as he usually did when thoughtful. Time passed. Cohen and Warden talked. Lillehei casually, but clearly, outlined his thoughts, and gave Warden and Cohen the okay to look into the crazy possibility of using the cardiovascular system of one animal to sustain the life of another.

Meanwhile, Lewis, after sixty successful ASD repairs, was confident enough to try his first ventricular septal defect repair under hypothermia. Ventricular septal defects, or VSDs, were generally larger holes, lower in the heart, in the septum between the muscular ventricles. Lillehei cautioned his friend that hypothermia would not allow enough operating time for the procedure should it be anything but extremely straight forward. The edgy Lewis snapped back that Lillehei was not the only hot shot in the department and planned to forge ahead.

The conversation that began with Cohen's wife's pregnancy evolved into controlled cross-circulation, which was how Lillehei described his vision of the circulatory system of a second animal sustaining the circulation of the first. Firmly convinced that the time constraints of hypothermia had been taken to the limit, he had his team working flat out on this new system to buy more operating time. The idea was to clamp off the blood circulating to the "patient" dog's heart and lungs, while connecting tubes from the "donor" dog to receive the deoxygenated blood, clear it of carbon dioxide, replenish the oxygen content, and return it to the "patient" at a point beyond the heart. The "donor" would function as the heart and lungs of the "patient," providing normally oxygenated blood to the rest of the body, and the brain in particular. A single, external pump controlled the flow to and from the patient. The volume of flow was an important variable. Beginning with the minimal flow necessary to sustain life, as determined by Cohen's azygos flow experiments, the volume of oxygenated blood flowing to the "patient" animal was gradually increased. Ultimately, three to five times azygos's flow was determined to be the magic volume for uncomplicated patient survival.

It was a brilliant scheme. After stumbling at the start, the team found a rhythm, and were able to sustain the animals on cross-circulation, disconnect them, and revive them normally. Then Lillehei added another variable to their experiments. Having mastered the technique of cross-circulation, they surgically created ventricular septal defects and repaired them to mimic what they intended to do for their young patients.

By the fall of 1953, Lillehei, Warden, and Cohen had sixteen consecutive successes hooking dogs to cross-circulation, creating VSDs, repairing the VSDs, and waking up normal, active animals.

Lillehei was confident in the procedure. The post-operative dogs were cured of their surgically created heart defects and appeared healthy, and he was preparing to make his case for bringing the procedure to the operating room. In a conversation with Paul Dwan, the pediatric cardiologist at the Variety Heart Hospital, the issue of the mental capacity of the animals post cross-circulation arose. Brain damage was, after all, the dreaded complication of oxygen deprivation, and the fact that the postoperative dogs wagged their tails, ate well, and played normally was not comforting enough.

Dwan proposed a unique experiment. As the son of a founder of 3M, Dwan was heir to a fortune. He was influential, philanthropic, and could have lived a life of total leisure. But doing nothing was not his style, and he was interested in the project for a number of reasons. Having suffered childhood rheumatic fever before the antibiotic age, he was afflicted with heart valve disease so prevalent in survivors. Although his rheumatic heart had somewhat hampered him, it was not disabling. He was not only very active, but had become one of the first pediatric cardiologists in the nation. The combination of his profession and his family wealth enabled him to wield considerable power at the Variety Heart Hospital, the nation's first institution solely devoted to heart patients.

Dwan was an avid bird hunter and bred and trained excellent, working, golden retrievers for that purpose. Field hunting dogs are trained to respond immediately to commands, and Dwan's dogs were prize-winning field trial dogs, among the best in the county. Watching the repeated success of Lillehei's cross-circulation experiments, Dwan suggested using a pair of his exquisitely trained dogs to test the theory of whether cross-circulation caused unrecognized brain damage. Though they obviously couldn't speak or take a post-operative IQ test, the retained ability to respond to multiple commands might help convince skeptics that the procedure spared the brain. The thirty minutes of cross-circulation time sustained by the dogs was twice that expected to be necessary for human surgery. Each of Dwan's retrievers awoke quickly and was soon back in the field responding perfectly. Having Paul Dwan in his corner was a big plus for Lillehei. With sixteen consecutive lab successes and an influential ally, he believed his case was solid.

By late fall of 1953, Lillehei was fully convinced that the next step forward in open-heart surgery was controlled cross-circulation. The remarkably simple apparatus he constructed consisted of an agricultural milk pump that drove blood through beer hoses at pre-calculated rates. The pump was an inexpensive piece of farm equipment, and the plastic beer tubing was both transparent so that air bubbles could be seen, and cheap enough to replace and sterilize for each case.

Lillehei made it known to the chief that he wanted his chance. Wangensteen, too, had his doubts that hypothermia was the answer to more complicated surgery, but he denied Lillehei's impassioned requests to bring his procedure to the operating room. Despite Lewis and Wangensteen not sharing the warmest of relationships, Lewis was the first man in the world to succeed at open-heart surgery, and he had earned the chance to try his hand at the next step.

It was unlike Lillehei to pressure Wangensteen, but he pushed. Wangensteen held his ground, and as word circulated through the department, relations became strained between Lillehei and his old friend, Lewis. For Lillehei, it was never personal. He was so confident of his case that he had preemptively identified a candidate already hospitalized at Variety. For Lewis, it had become personal. He was angry. He had the world's strongest record of heart surgery success, and he would not give way. Wangensteen strongly supported Lewis's right to try. Lillehei may have been the favored son, but only failure could take Lewis out of the picture.

With Wangensteen's blessing, Lewis moved ahead and operated on two children diagnosed with VSDs under hypothermia. Neither case went well. The first preoperative diagnosis had been incorrect. The defect was more complicated than the seven minutes allowed, and the child died. The second diagnosis of VSD was correct. Lewis operated and Lillehei assisted. Glancing at the clock, and drenched in perspiration, Lewis wasn't getting the job done and he was running out of time. Lillehei offered to take over. Frustrated and angry with himself, Lewis refused. He kept control until the end and left the operating room to personally deliver the terrible news to the parents.

Dejected and self-doubting, the thoughtful, intellectual Lewis shut down to lick his wounds. Wangensteen then threw his full support to Lillehei. He withdrew Lewis's research funding, passed it to Lillehei, and within a year had banished John Lewis, the first man to perform open-heart surgery, to a teaching position at an affiliated hospital.

★　★　★　★　★

The story of Lewis and Lillehei had never been one of outright competition, certainly not in Lillehei's eyes. Their friendship had been long standing and deep. Unlikely roommates and friends, each man could see the best in the other and remain supportive while working in the atmosphere of "friendly competition" fostered by Wangensteen. Closest friends through medical school, as newlywed surgical residents, they socialized as couples as well. It was a time of heavy drinking, hard work, and late nights. Though both bound by a strong work ethic, their styles differed so greatly that they could be expected to totally repel or attract one another. Sharing an office, they barely exchanged a word, but that was their normal. The cynical, complicated Lewis read widely, and found peace in classical music, and painting. Lillehei, a lover of jazz, enjoyed his music with multiple martinis at the Parker House. His reading was primarily work-related, and though he lacked self-doubt or introspection, he was magnanimous, and totally guileless.

CHAPTER SEVEN

WALT LILLEHEI

Clarence Walton Lillehei, Walt to everyone who knew him, was born in Minneapolis on October 23, 1918. His father was a successful dentist, and the family worked hard and lived well. A good student, inner-directed, mechanically gifted, curious, adventuresome, handsome, and very shy, Lillehei was educated entirely locally. He graduated with honors from the University of Minnesota and was elected to the Alpha Omega Alpha honor society at the medical school. He met and romanced Kaye Lindberg when he was an intern and she a nursing student at the University. Kaye had been dating someone else, who had already gone off to war. She had been immediately attracted to Walt's good looks and piercing, steel-blue eyes, but it was his single-minded devotion to his patients, and his unusual empathy for them that won her over. They were seeing each other exclusively by the time he completed his internship in June of 1942. Like the other young men of his generation, Lillehei enlisted in the army. Before shipping out, he and Kaye became engaged to be married.

As an army surgeon, Lillehei served first in North Africa, and then heroically in the bloody battlefield at Anzio in Italy, where he commanded a mobile army surgical hospital (MASH) and was awarded the bronze star for meritorious service in a combat zone. He was also briefly a prisoner of war after blindly following orders and attempting to take over a German field hospital still occupied by the enemy.

For the three years he was away, Lillehei wrote to Kaye as often as he could, always expressing his deep love for her. In Rome, after the horror of Anzio, Kaye may have been in his thoughts, but Lillehei carried R&R to the extreme. It would be a precedent he would follow for decades.

With three years of experience commanding a surgical unit, he was a seasoned administrator who longed to be a surgeon. Returning to Minneapolis, he showed up at the offices of the department of surgery at the University of Minnesota in the uniform of a Lieutenant Colonel. The department had been his home as an intern before the war, and the place to which he had dreamed of returning. Lillehei was directed to the office of Richard Varco, the senior surgeon in charge of the residency training program. Varco, with whom he had been acquainted as an intern, quickly deflated his aspirations by producing a list of returning trainees who had precedence for the few positions available.

Strong willed to begin with, Lillehei had been steeled by three years of war and was not about to accept rejection. Somehow, he secured an audience with Wangensteen, who was impressed with him, and he was hired on the spot. Given a white lab coat belonging to Varco that had been hanging nearby, he was taken on rounds by the chief and introduced to his new home. Department of surgery legend has it that after seeing the young Lieutenant Colonel he had just dismissed making ward rounds wearing Varco's own lab coat over his uniform, Varco never wore a lab coat again.

In January of 1946, Lillehei began his residency. He worked on the surgical wards and in the operating rooms, learning the very basics of his craft. It was exactly where he wanted to be. He and Kaye were married later that year, and soon had their daughter, Kimberly. The first two grinding residency years were followed by a year in the lab, and with no further surgical experience, he was appointed chief resident. It was hardly the sort of lengthy training demanded by the establishment where residencies would span five to seven years. But Wangensteen was first and foremost a research scientist whose attitude prioritized thinking and innovation above technique. Lillehei entered his chief residency short on experience and long on imagination and desire to learn.

During his chief resident year, Lillehei noticed a painless, pea-sized lump in front of his left ear. He was totally consumed with his responsibilities in the hospital and his young family and thought little of it. Finally, asking Wangensteen's advice when it persisted unchanged, he was convinced to have it excised. The tumor appeared to be within the parotid gland, and Wangensteen enlisted a skilled head and neck surgeon to remove it. The parotid gland, located in the cheek in front of the ear and below the earlobe, can be envisioned as a tortilla, folded over and containing the facial nerve. This is the motor nerve for the facial muscles. Damage to a branch of the nerve will weaken or paralyze portions of the face and turn facial expressions as simple as smiling into contortions. Injury to branches of the nerve can make the eyelid or mouth droop, mimicking Bell's palsy. Tumors of the parotid gland are traditionally treated with excision of at least a lobe of the gland itself, all the while keeping the nerve in sight and out of harm's way—tricky stuff demanding special care.

Lillehei underwent surgery in February, emerged unscathed, and was shortly back at work. The pathologist's report on the tumor was sent to Wangensteen, who was alarmed at the highly unusual diagnosis of lymphosarcoma of the parotid gland. This was a serious cancer with a negligible survival rate. Wangensteen sent slides and specimens to a number of major cancer centers including Memorial-Sloan Kettering, Columbia Presbyterian in New York, and the nearby Mayo Clinic. All confirmed the diagnosis, offering the pessimistic prognosis of five year survival from 5 percent to 25 percent. Even after all the opinions were in, Wangensteen, the man who believed in early, radical surgery, postponed telling Lillehei until he finished his residency. That would be in late May or June.

Wangensteen had big plans for his young protégé and had already posted prominently on the following year's assignment board: Dr. Lillehei, consultant specialist in open-heart surgery, a discipline that existed only in the laboratory, and in Wangensteen's imagination.

Just before Memorial Day of 1950, Wangensteen called Lillehei to his office, which was not at all unusual. Not having given much thought to the surgery for months, Lillehei was shocked by the bad news. Wangensteen proposed additional surgery. Lillehei listened and said little. He thanked Wangensteen without agreeing to the surgery and went to the library and began reading extensively on the subject. What he read did little to comfort him. After spending the day absorbing what he could about his situation, he went home to address it with Kaye. Lillehei filled her in on what he had learned in his crash course, and they discussed it into the night.

With no apparent option, he agreed to the extensive surgery Wangensteen had proposed. By the following week, a high-powered surgical team had been organized to deal with what Wangensteen had believed to be a life threatening situation. With ultimate confidence in his mentor, Lillehei underwent a ten hour operation requiring numerous surgeons and nine units of blood. The resident staff rallied behind their colleague. Those who could donated blood. Others volunteered to help in surgery. Everyone read up on the disease. Few had expected it to end well. Lillehei said nothing.

★ ★ ★ ★ ★

Wangensteen was generally known to be a particularly aggressive cancer surgeon. Many considered him so excessively aggressive that the running dark joke was that Wangensteen hated cancer so much because it killed more patients than he did.

Under Wangensteen's direct orders, the remainder of the parotid gland was removed, along with a left radical neck dissection encompassing removal of the major muscles and lymph nodes of the neck, along with a sternal splitting incision to remove the lymph node chains in the chest. It was super radical surgery for a cancerous node with no indication of spread. Wangensteen believed it warranted in the face of extremely malignant disease.

The surgery was a violent attack on glands, muscles, nerves, and blood vessels followed by radiation, and the post-operative period was painful and complicated for Lillehei. A week after surgery, the extensive wound on his chest became infected.

Areas of pus accumulated in the sternal incision requiring drainage and debridement, an aggressive type of surgical cleaning and removal of infected, damaged tissue. John Lewis and Richard Varco came to the Lillehei apartment after work each day to perform the unpleasant task.

Weak from surgery, radiation, infection, and blood loss, Lillehei was condemned to a summer in his small, duplex apartment. His discomfort was compounded by an unusually steamy, wet June. Temperatures topped out above 94 degrees, there was no air conditioning for relief, and he was too fatigued for excursions. Lillehei read very little, and television provided his primary diversion. That summer, the major league all-star game was televised for the first time, and baseball games, western movies, and variety shows were his entertainment through the long evenings until the test patterns replaced broadcasting. Sometimes he simply sat quietly alone doing nothing.

Kaye, acting as both wife and nurse, tried to be with her husband every moment she wasn't tending to their young daughter. With some difficulty, she managed to encourage nightly steak dinners to rebuild his strength, but she was unsuccessful in discouraging the martinis he shared with his visiting coworkers. Kaye worried as the dynamic young surgeon she married withdrew into an unaccustomed depression as he watched his world move on without him. Beyond generalized weakness from surgery and radiation, the most debilitating issue was the infected chest wound, which healed very slowly. Four months passed before Lillehei was strong enough to return to work.

The summer of 1950 had been unkind. His skeletonized left neck, and the scar coursing from his cheek onto his chest, were permanent reminders of the radical surgery he had endured. But he was alive. He had survived the war, seen its horrors firsthand, and now endured a horror of his own. At thirty-two, he had no idea if he would be among the one in four who survived the disease for five years—and then what? Iconoclastic, and ambitious to begin with, he had become increasingly unlike his coworkers. Lillehei was a finely tuned young man in a hurry, and for good reason.

Upon his return to work, Lillehei was officially a member of the senior staff, but technically junior to his contemporary, John Lewis. Like Lewis, Lillehei began his clinical practice, continued his laboratory work, and prepared for his dissertation for his doctorate in surgery. Both Lewis and Lillehei were becoming more technically adept as they moved up in the ranks of senior surgeons. Other young surgeons not enrolled in the combined residency and advanced degree program found Lillehei seriously lacking technically. Operative surgery is a practiced craft. Exposure and repetition are prerequisites for the development of skill and surgical judgement. Lillehei was fully aware of what he lacked. With innate ability and self-confidence, and not at all embarrassed, he would ask his juniors to teach him a procedure and rapidly become its master. While his intellectual interest focused on the possibilities of open-heart surgery, his work was general surgery, consultant in open-heart surgery, or not.

★　★　★　★　★

In September of 1952, Lillehei had been happy for Lewis's great success. His persistence in pursuing cross-circulation into the operating room was simply because he was certain that operating under hypothermia had taken open-heart surgery to the limits of its usefulness. Something better was needed to allow time for more complicated procedures. Lillehei had found it in cross-circulation. He had proven his point in the laboratory, but the worrisome ingredient that hung over cross-circulation was the potential risk to the individual providing circulating, oxygenated blood.

As he prepared to go forward, word circulated beyond the department of surgery, and not everyone saw it in a positive light. Wangensteen encouraged a visiting lecturer, Willis Potts, a prominent Chicago pediatric surgeon, to visit Lillehei's research laboratory. After witnessing a successful cross-circulation procedure, Potts told the expectant Lillehei that he would go down in history—and after a pregnant pause—as the first surgeon to have 200 percent mortality in a single operation. If Lillehei was any more than mildly surprised, he didn't show it, and he certainly was not dissuaded. He simply smiled and pushed forward.

Lewis had reached the limits of his procedure and was pushed from the stage. Gibbon initially succeeded with his heart-lung bypass machine, lost two children on the table, and quit. And so, in March of 1954, it was Lillehei's turn.

The ensuing months, tragic and elating in turn, marked the true beginning of open-heart surgery as a far reaching accepted surgical specialty with reproducible results. Once at the helm, Lillehei seemed to take giant steps on a monthly basis. Though Lillehei remains the least known of the pioneers in the field, it was he who made it happen. The others: Christiaan Barnard, Denton Cooley, Michael DeBakey, and Norman Shumway, each to the man, considered Walt Lillehei to have been the father of open-heart surgery. But his ascendence to that pedestal would be marred by elements worthy of Greek tragedy.

CHAPTER EIGHT

GREGORY GLIDDEN

G regory Glidden, the youngest of Lyman and Frances Glidden's ten children, had been fragile since birth. By six weeks of age, he had already been hospitalized with a respiratory infection. Over the next several months, he was hospitalized repeatedly with pneumonia, fatigue, and a significant heart murmur, which ultimately led to the diagnosis of an atrial septal, or ventricular septal defect.

Frances Glidden didn't need to be told. She had recognized the loud murmur, the symptoms, and the thrusting movements of his chest with each heartbeat. It was a pattern she had seen in her daughter, LaDonnah, who had only recently died from congenital heart disease. The Gliddens were encouraged by their family doctor to return to University Hospital where they were told a surgeon named John Lewis had been successfully repairing atrial septal defects.

Lyman Glidden worked the Mesabi iron range, the largest iron ore mine in the country. The family lived in the company town of Hibbing, 207 miles north of Minneapolis. Life was hard, pay was low, and maintaining the large family was a constant struggle.

The whole idea of more heart disease terrified the Gliddens. The doctors at University Hospital had been unable to save their daughter. But baby Gregory was so obviously ill that despite their foreboding, they deputized the older children to mind their siblings and made the long trip to Minneapolis in their old car, hoping against hope that something could be done.

Gregory was seen by the pediatricians and cardiologists at the children's ward of the Variety Club Heart Hospital, the newest addition to the University Hospital complex. Funded by $1.5 million from the Variety Club, which had begun in the entertainment industry, it was the first hospital in the country devoted to treating heart disease. A modern, four story structure, the brightly decorated third floor was devoted to pediatric cardiology and included an auditorium where movies were screened on Friday nights. The fourth floor housed laboratories and a skyway that connected Variety to the second floor of University Hospital and the operating rooms. There, eight months old, Gregory was admitted for testing and treatment. An X-ray revealed an enlarged heart, an ECG and cardiac catheterization indicated a septal defect; probably a hole in the ventricular septum. It was a defect that had never been successfully corrected. The cardiologist offered some optimism and hope, saying they were working on it, and baby Gregory was sent home.

By December, Gregory's condition had deteriorated. Fatigued, he ate little, failed to gain weight, and suffered repeated respiratory infections. Just after Christmas, he was transferred from the local Hibbing hospital to the Variety Club Heart Hospital. Instead of meeting John Lewis, the celebrity surgeon they had expected, the Gliddens were introduced to Lillehei, whom they had never heard of. Lillehei patiently explained that he was working on a new procedure that promised enough operating time to fix Gregory's defect, that it was still experimental and had never been performed of a human patient. He was interested, and empathetic, and his quiet, unhurried manner impressed the Gliddens. Frances was already very pregnant yet again, and with Lyman at work, and nine children at home, Gregory was left at the children's ward of the hospital.

Days became weeks and months. Gregory passed his first birthday at the hospital. A happy child, he quickly became a favorite of the nurses. Despite constant attention and the best care, his physical condition remained unstable. Lillehei hoped for a healthy interlude to give the child a better chance at surgery, but the pneumonia continued to wax and wane unpredictably. Finally, Gregory seemed relatively healthy, and Lillehei was ready. He made his case as forcefully as possible, but at this point, Wangensteen, again citing Lewis's prior successes with atrial septal defects, insisted he be given his chance first. Lillehei was convinced that Lewis simply couldn't accomplish a difficult VSD repair in the seven or eight minute window afforded by hypothermia. He had pushed as far as he dared, and after being repeatedly denied, Lillehei assisted and waited, until, sadly, John Lewis failed in two attempts to correct a VSD, and it was his turn. His, and Gregory Glidden's.

The circumstances were more charged than usual, even in the electric world of introducing new procedures into the operating room. Gregory Glidden had been in the hospital for three months and was adored by all. Lillehei had seen him often enough to have well exceeded the normal bond of doctor patient relationship. In addition to the risks of the new procedure, Lewis, his closest friend, had had to fail in order for Lillehei to have his chance. That meant children had to die.

Fearing catastrophe, chief of medicine Cecil Watson and chief of pediatrics Irvine McQuarrie, immediately appealed to the hospital administrator to prevent the cross-circulation surgery from proceeding. Both men had been supportive of John Lewis. They had been proud of his successes and stung by his failures. Both believed in the surgical adventurism of cross-circulation, but the risk of losing a patient, and the human oxygenator, could deal a staggering blow to the university. The offhand dismissal of the concept by Willis Potts had further fanned the flames. But it all made simple sense to Lillehei. Cross-circulation had worked smoothly and consistently in the lab, he was sure of his groundwork, and he ignored the naysayers. Wangensteen was in his corner, and Wangensteen was the only authority to whom Lillehei answered.

From December through late March, Gregory Glidden weathered several episodes of pneumonia. He was more than a year old and weighed only eleven pounds, half the weight of the average boy his age. Gregory was not making progress and seemed as strong as he was going to be, facing the considerable toll of his heart defect. As surgery neared, Lillehei was busy preparing himself. He studied anatomy books and occasional autopsy specimens trying to feel at home with all variations of human pathologic anatomy. Needing to know all he possibly could, he decided to take advantage of a unique opportunity two hours south, at the Mayo Clinic. There, the well-known pathologist Jesse Edwards ruled over the world's largest known collection of human hearts—autopsy specimens collected over decades and stored in formalin filled pickle barrels.

Lillehei had recently treated himself to a flashy Buick Roadmaster convertible, which he loved to drive. Along with Varco, and his lab crew, Warden and Cohen, the foursome made a trip to Mayo and spent the day examining the endless array of preserved hearts. Each heart had been cut open and carefully tagged, displaying every variation of pathologic anatomy. What he did not want to find at surgery were surprises. The field trip made the team acutely aware of the infinite variety of defects they might encounter, and the sudden awareness of how little they knew rattled as much as informed them. Inside the closed car, with the pervasive smell of formalin still surrounding them, the trip home was filled with equal doses of optimistic planning and black humor. But Lillehei felt better prepared and confident.

He chose March 26, 1954, for surgery.

Typically, operating schedules are organized in the late afternoon prior to the following day's surgery. On the morning of March 25, twelve hours before it was scheduled, indication of the use of controlled cross-circulation was typed, mimeographed, and posted, but rumors of the proposed surgery had already made the rounds. Watson, McQuarrie, and the hospital administrator confronted Wangensteen, who heard them out but refused to back down. Lillehei would have his chance.

After a full day of surgery that ran well into the evening, Lillehei returned to his office to find a handwritten note from Wangensteen.

Dear Walt,

By all means, go ahead!
Good luck.

O.H.W.

Lyman Glidden had the same O+ blood type as Gregory, and he volunteered to have his heart and lungs provide oxygenated blood to his son, whose own heart and lungs would be excluded from circulation for the surgery.

At 6:00 a.m., Lyman Glidden was rolled on a stretcher into operating room number two and transferred onto an operating table. Gregory was carried into the room and placed on the second operating table in the room. Meanwhile, Lillehei was in another operating room performing a routine hernia repair as if it were just another day at the office.

Cross-circulation utilized vessels in Lyman's groin to connect to his son. To facilitate this, Lyman had been positioned on his back, at about the level of his son's head. Gregory was on his back as well. Two anesthesiologists attended to each patient. Each was put to sleep with intravenous sodium pentothal, after which endotracheal breathing tubes were inserted. Cyclopropane, an anesthetic more manageable, but equally as explosive as ether, was pumped from its cylinder to the patient through a black rubber reservoir bag that the anesthesiologist squeezed rhythmically at fifteen times a minute. Warden and Varco made the circulatory connections while Morley Cohen ran the blood pump.

The setup was astoundingly simple and direct. Tubes collected deoxygenated blood from Gregory's venae cavae via a catheter in his femoral vein, and delivered it to Lyman's femoral vein, through which it flowed to the right side of Lyman's heart to his lungs. Here, it was oxygenated, returned to Lyman's heart, and pumped out via his aorta to his arteries. The femoral artery in Lyman's groin was connected by catheter to Gregory's left subclavian artery where it arose from his aorta, beyond his heart. Thus, freshly oxygenated blood was delivered to

Gregory's brain. Between father and son was the sigma motor pump, a simple device used primarily in food manufacturing. The pump squeezed the incoming and outgoing tubes to propel liquids, in this case, the blood in the two tubes. One in, one out, and both at the same rate. The whole pumping apparatus was external, so there were no sterility concerns beyond the interior of the tubing. Morley Cohen calculated the pumping at forty cubic centimeters of blood per kilogram of body weight for Gregory. He would man the pump and watch the dial. The simple pump did the rest. The most unusual member of the team was a secretary armed with a pencil and note pad to record the exact time spent on each segment of the procedure.

Lillehei opened the baby's chest with a long, transverse incision, and spread the ribs. He and Richard Varco gently wrapped cloth surgical tapes around the inferior and superior venae cavae, inserted plastic catheters, secured them with the tapes, and connected the transparent beer hose from the catheter in Lyman's femoral artery into Gregory's subclavian artery. Lillehei indicated he was ready to begin.

"Time Zero" Lillehei said calmly. Gregory's heart and lungs were no longer necessary to keep him alive.

Lillehei had a large head lamp he'd borrowed from an ENT surgeon strapped to his forehead. He said nothing else. Intent and direct as always, he never spoke unnecessarily in the operating room. Briefly contemplating the open chest, he made a one inch incision through the wall of the right ventricle and stared into the interior of Gregory's heart. There was little enough azygos blood back flow to be controlled by Varco with suction. Lillehei struggled to focus the light through the tiny hole in the lemon-sized heart and was momentarily lost. He blindly inserted his index finger into the ventricle and felt the hole in the septum. With Varco working to gently hold the incision open with small retractors, and free of blood with the suction cannula, Lillehei finally managed to see the defect. He grasped the edges of the hole in the septum with his forceps and quickly sutured them together under direct vision. Checking the repair, he added one more suture, signaled Varco to withdraw the suction cannula, and allowed the heart to fill with blood. When the ventricle overflowed, he sewed the incision in the right ventricle closed.

"Pump off."

The heart had been open for twelve and a half minutes.

Lillehei and Varco smiled above their masks, reached across the table, shook bloody, gloved hands, and looked up to the observation gallery where Wangensteen stood and led the applause.

The entire operation had taken nineteen minutes and Gregory was breathing on his own, circulating his own well-oxygenated blood, and uttering healthy postoperative cries.

In the absence of intensive care units and post-surgery recovery areas, patients recovering from surgery returned to their rooms. Gregory was brought across the bridge to his room in the Variety Club Heart Hospital, where he was placed in a croup tent supplied with cool oxygenated mist. The nurses watching over him were fully trained in the care he would need, and he did well. Neither father nor son appeared to suffer any ill effects from the surgery. Lillehei was quietly elated.

Visiting his young patient several times a day quickly became Lillehei's routine. Everything went well through the end of the first week, until Gregory refused food and developed a fever. He became lethargic, rallied, then became obviously ill again. Twice in the next days, Lillehei rushed to his bedside, once bringing him to surgery where an emergency tracheostomy was performed. This allowed the nurses to suction his trachea and provide a direct route for oxygen. Twice, he managed to bring Gregory back from the brink, but the child's breathing was rapid, his lungs became congested, and his fever persisted. Despite antibiotics and respiratory care, pneumonia had recurred. Gregory continued to weaken. On the eleventh post-operative day, despite heroic efforts at cardiac resuscitation, Gregory Glidden died.

Everyone was heartbroken. The boy was doted on by the nursing staff and had become a beloved member of the hospital family. Lillehei had made surgical history for a moment, and then he hadn't, and Frances and Lyman Glidden had lost another child to a ventricular septal defect.

The Gliddens had been advised of Gregory's critical condition, but sadly didn't arrive from Hibbing until shortly after their son had died. Lillehei, who had waited for them, offered heartfelt condolences. The sadness he shared with them had been obvious. When he requested permission for an autopsy to determine exactly what had transpired, the Gliddens agreed.

Later that day, Lillehei, in scrubs, a surgical cap, and a mask hanging on his chest, walked alone down the stairs to the morgue. The pathologist had nearly completed his work. He turned to Lillehei and handed him the tiny heart. Lillehei held it in his cupped hands and stared at it without speaking. Then, he gently placed Gregory's heart on the stainless steel table, and with a surgical scalpel cut into it, laying open the ventricle.

Had it had been humanly possible to stand in the morgue holding the heart of a recently deceased child and be happy, what Lillehei saw through his tears had made him happy. The site of his repair was completely healed. The operation had been a success. The autopsy showed that Gregory Glidden's ventricular septal defect was cured. He had died of pneumonia.

Carved in the single headstone marking the graves of LaDonnah and Gregory Glidden is the inscription, "His little heart changed the world."

CHAPTER NINE

SUCCESS MEETS CONFLICT

Lillehei shared the news vindicating both his team and Wangensteen. Though it didn't mitigate the sadness of losing Gregory, he had been right, and he intended to move forward. His detractors in the hospital were unmoved by the autopsy findings. They held fast to their ethical objections and intended to prevent any further attempts at cross-circulation. While the arguments continued, two suitable candidates were quietly identified and waited in the wings. When Lillehei learned that Watson and McQuarrie both planned to be out of town for medical conferences, he scheduled the next two surgeries for April 20 and 23. The patients were four-year-old Bradley Mehrman and five-year-old Pamela Schmidt. Both had been diagnosed with ventricular septal defects, and despite multiple illnesses, both were stable, and far healthier than Gregory Glidden had been.

The plan was to complete both surgeries even if the first child didn't survive. Lillehei was certain his path was correct. "When something has to be done, it's got to be done," he repeated.

But both operations went smoothly, and both children were discharged home several days after surgery. When the good news filtered down from the operating suite, the same hospital administrators who had attempted to block the surgery now arranged elaborate press conferences for Lillehei and his team. Although he was a flashy dresser, Lillehei was a reticent speaker, and he blandly described the procedure for the newsreel cameras. Warden and Cohen explained the cross-circulation hookup and the operation of the pump, and then, to add a touch of showmanship, Pamela Schmidt and her parents spoke to the assembled press, who dubbed her the queen of hearts. The press conference made it onto an NBC news medical report, and it was Lillehei who was seen as a hero.

A few weeks later, at a surgical meeting in Montreal, Lillehei had Warden present their laboratory work on cross-circulation in dogs. The audience included most of those who had struggled unsuccessfully to conquer open-heart surgery as well as young surgeons anxious to join the party. Since the talk was about experimental surgery, it didn't arouse much interest. Then, Lillehei stood and shocked the audience with a report on the first three surgical cases using controlled cross-circulation on children. When he finished his short presentation, there was absolute silence. Not even polite applause. Young men like Denton Cooley were excited by the news, but the sight of this brash fellow in a checked jacket, alligator shoes, and gold watch did nothing to soften the response among the older, conservative, early pioneers. Robert Gross was icy in his silence. Gibbon, who had lost three of four patients using his bypass machine, first cited his one success, then pointed out that there must be some risk to the healthy donor in cross-circulation and suggested they seek a method that didn't pose that risk. Lillehei laughingly whispered to Cohen that if Gibbon didn't like it then they must be right.

In the next four months, Lillehei succeeded in six of eight operations. Determined to hold course, he continued working at what was, for him at the time, a furious pace, accepting children for surgery who would otherwise have been doomed.

Over the course of a year, Lillehei used controlled cross-circulation for forty-five operations. Each was a potentially lifesaving operation on a desperately ill child. Only twenty-eight lived, a survival rate of 62 percent. But, twenty-eight children were saved where there would have been none only a year earlier. However, the loss of seventeen frail, young children, no matter that they had no other hope, did not make Lillehei popular. That fall, after a particularly tragic series of cases in which he lost six of seven patients, the stoic Lillehei became morose. There was talk of discontinuing the program, and to make matters worse, Lillehei had overheard the floor nurses refer to him as a murderer.

Despite his steely self-assurance and otherworldly ability to ignore professional criticism, this hurt him, and for the first time, the unshakeable Lillehei began to doubt himself. Losing six of seven patients was unthinkable. His stalwart supporters in the hospital, as well as his wife Kaye at home, repeatedly pointed out the obvious: he saved the lives of more than half of the children that would otherwise have died. In fact, he was the only person in the world offering these children the chance to live. Lillehei ultimately came around as his numbers improved. And as the numbers improved, the surgical problems he took on became increasingly more complex.

Even Lillehei had known at the outset that mechanical bypass was the ultimate goal, but two jolting episodes made him look more immediately in directions beyond cross-circulation. In the first case, a donor mother suffered cardiac arrest after being disconnected from cross-circulation. In a dramatic moment, Lillehei slashed open her chest, massaged her heart, and resuscitated her. The woman bore no ill effects beyond a scar across her chest, but the baby died on the second postoperative day. In all, it had been a disaster.

In the second incident, while putting the donor mother to sleep prior to cross-circulation, the anesthesiologist inadvertently delivered an air embolus into her intravenous line. The operation was aborted, but the woman suffered permanent, debilitating brain damage. Although Lillehei was not directly at fault, he advised the husband, an air force officer, to sue both him and the hospital to recover the costs of permanent nursing care from their insurance carrier. Once the lawyers got involved, a number of accusations were leveled at Lillehei, including lack of informed consent, and a very large settlement was demanded. The charges were vigorously defended, and the case was dismissed from Federal Court. It would not be the only time Lillehei faced a judge in Federal Court.

★　★　★　★　★

Through the summer of 1954, Lillehei was the only surgeon in the country doing open-heart cases. He was a giant step ahead of where his pioneering friend, John Lewis, had been, and he was ready to take on the most complicated of congenital heart lesions, a complex of multiple abnormalities called the tetralogy of Fallot. At a time when most people knew nothing about heart defects, and even less about heart surgery, many knew the term tetralogy of Fallot. Though complicated to explain, and seemingly impossible to correct, it was the lesion that brought the world to believe that heart surgery was possible. All the excitement began in 1944, with an extra-cardiac, palliative correction that made Alfred Blalock, the Johns Hopkins surgeon, and Helen Taussig, the pediatric cardiologist, world famous.

The tetralogy was initially described as early as the seventeenth century, and ultimately named after Étienne-Louis Arthur Fallot, the French physician who described it in detail in 1888. The complex requires study for even knowledgeable physicians. It consists of pulmonary stenosis, causing reduced flow of oxygenated blood from the lungs to the left atrium; ventricular septal defect, which allows oxygenated blood to reenter the right ventricle instead of being fully pumped out via the aorta; right ventricular hypertrophy; and an overriding aorta, which allows blood from both ventricles, oxygenated and unoxygenated, to enter the aorta.

The combined defects resulted in "blue babies," named for the deep blue cast of the children's lips and fingernails. Rounded or clubbed fingertips, failure to thrive, and fainting episodes on exertion make up the clinical syndrome. In severe cases, even the simple act of eating might cause all of the above. The long-term prognosis was awful, and few children with full-blown cases lived to adulthood.

On November 29, 1944, Blalock, chief of surgery at Johns Hopkins, and his team performed the first "blue baby" operation. The procedure was actually proposed by Helen Taussig, the pediatric cardiologist director of the children's hospital at Hopkins, who was a full partner in the endeavor.

The operation is based on the ductus arteriosus, an embryonic vessel that connects the pulmonary artery to the aorta in utero, bypassing the lungs. This is quite efficient in utero. Since there is no air to breathe, the lungs are unnecessary and the placenta delivers fully oxygenated blood to the embryo. By birth, or shortly after birth, the ductus arteriosus between the aorta and the pulmonary artery closes, and normal circulation through the lungs begins.

The idea for the operation came about because Taussig noticed that children with tetralogy of Fallot, whose ductus arteriosus remained open, had milder symptoms and lived longer than those whose ductus had closed. On that premise, she and Blalock devised an operation to create an artificial ductus by connecting the subclavian artery, a large artery that branches off the aorta, to the pulmonary artery. The actual surgical procedure was largely the work of Vivien Thomas, Blalock's black laboratory assistant, who was initially denied credit in the Jim Crow south of 1944.

In a child spared other cardiac defects a ductus arteriosus that remains open, or patent, after birth results in oxygenated blood from the high-pressure aorta, being pushed back into the lungs through the low-pressure pulmonary artery instead of fully nourishing the body. This causes children with a patent ductus to suffer symptoms of oxygen deprivation. Hence, after birth, it is physiologically important that the ductus is closed. In 1938, Robert Gross, a Boston surgeon, performed the first surgical closure of a patent's ductus arteriosus, essentially tying off the connection between the pulmonary artery and the aorta and completing what nature had forgotten to do. This too was an extra-cardiac operation, not in the heart, but around the heart. It was a much-heralded step forward, but not open-heart surgery.

Gross was among those who labored unsuccessfully with early attempts at open-heart techniques. He was a caustic critic of everyone but himself. When Blalock relieved the severity of the tetralogy by creating an artificial ductus arteriosus, Gross derided the accomplishment by saying, "I correct the ductus arteriosus, not create it."

But the operation improved the lives and longevity of children with tetralogy and created a worldwide sensation. Hailed as heart surgery, which it wasn't, it did put the idea of heart surgery into the public consciousness.

No further advances were made toward correcting the tetralogy for a decade. Then, in August of 1954, Lillehei made the giant leap of actually correcting a version of the tetralogy under cross-circulation. No one had ever before repaired the tetralogy in any form, but the monumental achievement didn't receive the professional acclaim he had expected. With his irreverent, blunt manner and unconventional thinking, Lillehei rubbed the senior surgeons the wrong way. Worse, he had succeeded where they had failed.

Among his heretical innovations, Lillehei used synthetic cloth patches to close VSDs. Foreign bodies had never been introduced into the heart before, and once again, a long-held rule had been proven wrong. The material he used, Ivalon, was relatively inert, and well tolerated, but for ease of handling reasons was soon replaced with Teflon. The patch idea made obvious sense. The VSD hole is often quite large, with attenuated, friable edges. Trying to close the hole side to side presented many problems, paramount among them was the deformity caused by successful closure; like cutting a circle of cloth out of a pant leg and discarding it, and then just sewing the gap closed. It doesn't work, or at least it doesn't look like a pant leg.

In repairing heart defects, the tension that sutures put on the tissue had to be considered. Too much tension risked tearing and destroying what remained of the septum. Patching defects with inert material solved both the deformity and tension issues. Success using patches on VSDs encouraged Lillehei to apply the same solution to the tissue deficient pulmonary artery, which was part of the tetralogy of Fallot. The patch increased the diameter of the attenuated pulmonary artery and allowed more blood flow to the lungs. The wisdom of these innovations is attested to by the fact that they remain to this day the procedure of choice. Lillehei's sensible but radical step opened the door to fashioning other artificial materials into heart valves and grafts.

In another moment of surgical ingenuity, Lillehei inserted an unconnected pulmonary artery directly into the right ventricle, without a pulmonary valve to prevent backflow. Postulating on the spot that the pulmonary system being a low-pressure system compared to the left side of the heart, he concluded that the valve was unnecessary. Not only was his logic correct, but his procedure has stood the test of time.

While all this was going on, Lillehei and company had not stopped looking at other schemes for bypassing the heart. One that had been tried elsewhere was the idea of using dog lungs as oxygenators. The lab experience had been to connect a dog's lung directly to its circulation, excluding the heart. And it was successful. Taken a step further, the self-oxygenating setup led to freshly harvesting dog lungs, purging them of blood by thoroughly washing them through with saline solution, suspending them in an oxygen rich container, and connecting them to a patient to bypass the heart and oxygenate the body. The setup was tried in a human experiment without any detectable side effects, and the idea ultimately found its way up to Lillehei, who thought it was worth a try. The first patient died after surgery, and although the process itself had proven its merit, Lillehei was not ready to abandon cross-circulation.

In August of 1954, Calvin Richmond, a thirteen-year-old Arkansas boy was run over by an ice wagon and suffered a traumatic ventricular septal defect. The boy was from a poor black family, the accident made the news, and the local community rallied behind him. Children raised money for his care, and he was flown to Minneapolis to see the now famous Lillehei, who volunteered his services free of charge. And then the problems began. Calvin's mother, who accompanied him, and whose blood type matched, refused to be anesthetized. Authorities reached out to the local prison for cross-circulation volunteers, but none were willing to have their blood intermixed with the blood of a Black boy. With no other choice, Lillehei decided to use the dog lungs. The operation went well. The VSD was closed, and Calvin recovered without incident and returned to Arkansas. After that resounding success, Lillehei used the dog lung apparatus a dozen times more with unpredictable results and went back to cross-circulation, all the while, looking for the safest way into the heart. He had made advance after advance in a tumultuous year, and he had just begun.

★　★　★　★　★

At a meeting in Philadelphia in May of 1955, Lillehei first reported on his use of a patch graft to close a VSD, as well as his technique for correcting the tetralogy of Fallot. The all-star audience included John Gibbon, who built the first bypass machine, Alfred Blalock, and Helen Taussig of blue baby operation fame.

After Lillehei's presentation, Blalock stood and admitted that he had not believed the tetralogy of Fallot could ever be surgically corrected. But the compliment ended there. Blalock went on to say that cross-circulation was not the ultimate answer, and that many other surgeons were using heart-lung bypass machines like the one built by Gibbon.

That cross-circulation was not the ultimate answer was true enough, even Lillehei knew that. But others around the country were not using bypass machines. In fact, the only heart-lung bypass machine in use at the time was at the Mayo Clinic. It was used by Lillehei's friend, John Kirklin, only twice, and only two weeks prior to the meeting. Blalock was either misinformed or anti-Lillehei.

While Lillehei still held the stage, the grey-haired visage of Blalock's partner, the fifty-seven-year-old Dr. Helen Taussig, rose, and to the shock of all present, began shouting, "This criminal must be stopped."

The auditorium filled with whispers and then went silent.

Whatever her beliefs and motivation, the outburst was unusual, totally out of order, and marked the end of the era of Blalock and Taussig as the saviors of babies with tetralogy of Fallot. They had been relegated to history books and hadn't yet known it.

Lillehei, of course, was unmoved. He ignored the outburst as though he hadn't heard it, and he stood by his monumental advances with cross-circulation. It had bought operative time when it was desperately needed, but he too knew it was an interim measure. Quietly, Lillehei and Richard DeWall were preparing to use their own bypass machine. They were busy with surgery by day and working with the machine at night. Preparing the presentation on tetralogy had taken time and caused them to delay the first clinical use of their own machine until May 13th, less than two weeks *after* the meeting. Having not yet used the apparatus for human surgery, Lillehei made no mention of it in his talks. Future plans were unproven. He was there to report on what he had already done, not what he hoped to do. Lillehei dealt with Taussig's diatribe in the same manner in which he dealt with the scorching comments of Gross, Gibbon, and Potts: he ignored them. He was moving on.

The DeWall-Lillehei bypass machine, about to be used clinically for the first time, was unlike anything seen before. The contrast with its predecessors staggered the imagination. It was a simple contraption that cost less than fifty dollars to make and would soon be available to all.

CHAPTER TEN

SOWING THE SEEDS

In June of 1955, barely a month after Taussig's banishment into obsolescence, Denton Cooley decided to see what was going on in Minnesota. He and Dan McNamara, a Baylor pediatric cardiologist, made the trip from Houston to Minneapolis together. The plan was to visit Lillehei, then drive down to Rochester to see John Kirklin at Mayo, and the modified Mayo–Gibbon heart–lung machine he had, by then, used several times.

Lillehei showed the visitors around the unit and the wards, and then surprised them with a quick preview of the heart–lung machine that Richard DeWall and he had devised. By this time, the contraption had already been used successfully for human surgery. For reasons he failed to explain, he was not planning to employ it at surgery the following day. The machine itself was an unimpressive tangle of coils, tubes, and a simple pump, all of which hung freely without benefit of a sleek container. Cooley circled it, asked a few questions about the bubble oxygenator, instantly understood it, and saw the beauty in its simplicity. McNamara saw a tangle of coils, tubes, and a milk pump.

On the evening before surgery, Lillehei hosted his guests for dinner at the Parker House. When they entered, the bartender greeted Lillehei enthusiastically, and asked if he wanted the usual. Lillehei nodded, pointed to his guests, and double martinis were delivered to each. The visitors quit at two doubles. They enjoyed good conversation and steak dinners. After dinner, Lillehei quickly went through two more double martinis. Soon, he and Cooley were dancing with the waitresses. Cooley and McNamara stumbled out at 1:00 a.m. and took a taxi to their hotel. Lillehei was having too much fun to leave.

Surgery was scheduled for the next morning at 9:00 a.m. Cooley and McNamara, a bit undone by the previous evening, had also been forced to share a room and a bed. They overslept, awoke confused, and in a panic, hurriedly dressed, and arrived at 9:30 a.m., rumpled, unshaven, and apologetic. And then they waited. No Lillehei. At 10:00 a.m., a sweaty Lillehei, looking much the worse for wear, arrived at the scrub sink, performed the ritual ten minute scrub, dried his hands with a sterile cotton towel, held his arms out for the sterile cotton gown, and pushed his hands into the gloves held in front of him. A nurse wiped his brow and snapped an amyl nitrite capsule under his nose. Lillehei shook his head from the fumes, greeted his visitors, leaned into the table, called "pump on," and performed a swift repair of a VSD under cross-circulation. Cooley was amazed. McNamara was horrified.

Their visit to the Mayo Clinic the following day was only ninety miles away, but in a different universe. Kirklin was a hospitable gentleman, and thoroughly professional, if a bit distant. He gave the full tour, and his staff of some fifty people who ran his laboratory and operated the Mayo-Gibbon heart-lung machine, were available for questions. Cooley and McNamara were welcomed as Kirklin's houseguests that evening, and after a glass of sherry and an early dinner with the family, the group took to their respective beds at 8:45 p.m. Cooley and McNamara were exhausted and hungover, and eagerly welcomed the early night.

The next morning, an operation performed using the complex heart-lung machine went off without a hitch, and the patient did well. McNamara was as impressed with Kirklin as he was put off by Lillehei. On the flight home to Houston, the pediatric cardiologist told Cooley, "You are not going to operate on any of my patients until you can duplicate what Dr. Kirklin and his team can do."

This put Cooley in a box. His boss, Michael DeBakey, had already made it clear there were no funds available for a one-hundred-thousand-dollar machine like the Mayo-Gibbon, nor would he support Cooley's efforts to acquire one.

Cooley had followed the events in Minneapolis closely. He had seen Kirklin's machine, but he knew that Lillehei had successfully used his own heart-lung machine seven times, and had, by that time, virtually abandoned cross-circulation, which had been off the table for Cooley from the moment he had his conversation with McNamara. Anxious to move forward, he pressed Lillehei for details and drawings, and Lillehei, as always, shared happily. As soon as Cooley knew the details, he enlisted two medical students and set about building his own DeWall-Lillehei device.

Lillehei had not arbitrarily concluded that he needed a heart-lung machine. It had always been the holy grail, but the versions he had seen were far too complicated, with too much room for error. It had to be simpler.

Lillehei, Warden, and Cohen had experimented with a number of ingenious systems in addition to the one that relied on azygos flow to oxygenate the brain, which never quite excited him enough. There was a trial in which five liters of oxygenated blood was slowly administered, and another using dog lungs in an oxygen container, which, despite the success with Calvin Richmond, was abandoned as unreliable. A number of ideas tried in the lab had not been original with Lillehei, who was not obsessed by being first at anything. He believed library research stifled the imagination and led to repetition of mistakes made by others, so even outrageous ideas were given a full hearing. He could go no further with controlled cross-circulation. Though it greatly increased the window of operating time and saved twenty-eight young lives, there had been a tragedy and a near tragedy, and the inherent risk to the donor remained too real.

Over the usual end of the week drinks with Warden and Cohen at the Parker House, interesting ideas regularly surfaced. Most were dismissed as too complex. They even touched on the ideas of screen oxygenators like Gibbons, and bubble oxygenators, which hadn't worked, looking for a new approach to old ideas. With a unique ability to collect information and disregard what didn't interest him, Lillehei continued to grind out ideas and file them away on index cards. Around the hospital, he was known for ignoring small talk and ideas that bored him. It didn't take much for him to be transported elsewhere. But when something struck him as right, he jumped on it and didn't let go. His instinct either opened his eyes and his mind or shut them down. There was no middle ground. It was a trait he carried into social situations. If he was disinterested, he shut down, much to the annoyance of individuals on the receiving end of what might be considered antisocial behavior. If he was interested, nothing else existed. This problem held his interest.

★ ★ ★ ★ ★

Early in 1954, Varco marched Richard DeWall into Lillehei's lab uninvited and carrying a plaster model of a heart valve he devised. Lillehei, who had already broken down the barriers against introducing foreign substances into the heart, was fascinated. But he was more interested in how DeWall's mind worked than the valve he was promoting.

DeWall was a general practitioner bored with stuffy noses and earaches. He wanted to be a surgeon and returned to his alma mater looking for a position. The residency program was overstaffed and underfunded, and his record at the medical school was undistinguished. Still, DeWall fit the mold of Lillehei's group of tinkerers. Lillehei wanted DeWall around, and in the absence of a residency position, an entry level spot was offered to him. DeWall jumped at the opportunity. Starting as an animal care worker, he soon became a part of the team in the laboratory and the operating room, running the pump and suggesting improvements. By then, the subject of oxygenators was a constant topic at the Parker House.

In September of 1954, Lillehei assigned DeWall the task of devising a simple oxygenator that could become their heart-lung machine.

The method DeWall and Lillehei came up with was a six-foot-tall bubble oxygenator that ingeniously side stepped the problem of air bubbles with a simple solution. The oxygen would be bubbled into a blood-filled container, producing large, easily visible and easily burst bubbles. The foam head on top of the blood reservoir would be dispersed by a type of silicone used in the dairy industry, and then, as the blood flowed down a five-foot spiral of beer tubing, the remaining bubbles would escape through the surface of the blood before it was pumped back into the patient.

The Rube Goldberg contraption, with its beer tubes, corks, and laboratory beaker stands looked like a high school science project, and appeared laughably amateurish next to the Mayo-Gibbon behemoth. But it worked. The parts were easily sterilized and easily replaced. It was simple to operate and it cost virtually nothing.

As Cooley had observed, Lillehei and Kirklin, just ninety miles apart in Minnesota, were worlds apart in demeanor and approach, but their goal was the same and they were in constant contact. They were, after all, the only open-heart surgeons in the world.

Kirklin, a very skilled surgeon, albeit one with a statistician's outlook, respected Lillehei's work. The two men shared this mutual respect in public and argued their cases in private. Cooley knew this. They represented the future, and he wanted into the select group. Stymied by the adamant refusal of his Houston pediatric cardiology colleague to refer patients for cross-circulation and by DeBakey's refusal to fund the one-hundred-thousand-dollar Kirklin machine, Cooley was delighted to see the new bubble oxygenator, and even happier to hear that it worked. It was the answer to his problems as well.

Lillehei had great faith in the simple machine. Barely two weeks after Helen Taussig had called him a criminal, he was using it successfully in the operating room. Not every child with severe congenital heart disease survived, nor had they with cross-circulation, but the machine functioned flawlessly. As usual, when Lillehei presented his newest advance, the old guard found reasons to denigrate it. There were whispers and asides calling him reckless, a cowboy, and a liar. To make matters worse, a number of surgeons who saw the simple machine altered it, and after their "improvements," found it lacking. Losing dog after dog to air emboli and hemorrhage, they blamed their failures on the machine. None, however, had used the simple machine as designed, and none had ultimately used it for human surgery. Contrary to the conventional wisdom of the time, it was harder to sustain dogs on the heart-lung machine than humans. As the far-flung experimenters condemned the DeWall-Lillehei machine, its failure to find popular use seemed preordained.

Deaf to the criticism, Lillehei continued to use his machine with great success. When he finally presented his results at a meeting almost two years later, the uninitiated, untalented, and old fashioned shouted him down. Lillehei had become accustomed to this sort of reception. He was not one of them. At meetings, Lillehei was where the party was, not where the professors were. His detractors saw someone unlike themselves. Someone whose unconventional ideas leap frogged the status quo and didn't pander to them. Proud of the success of his bypass machine, he again rose to face a crowd prepared to deride rather than listen and support him. And once again, they shouted him down.

Finally, Cooley stood up to speak above the din, "I have operated on over two hundred patients with DeWall-Lillehei oxygenators and have not encountered any problems from the heart-lung machine." Nothing more needed to be said. Not only was that the end of the derision, it also marked the entry of Denton Arthur Cooley into the pantheon of master heart surgeons. This cardiac cowboy also dressed the part, wearing lizard boots and the occasional Stetson. He was thirty-six years old and already the busiest cardiac surgeon in the world.

Years later, when Cooley's star was at its apex, he summed up the journey by saying, "If heart surgery was a picnic, Walt Lillehei brought the can opener."

CHAPTER ELEVEN

PROBLEMS FROM SUCCESS

By 1957, Cooley was using the bypass machine on nearly a daily basis. His boss, Michael DeBakey wasn't on board yet and didn't see the ship leaving any time soon. He was already well known for his work with aortic aneurysms and wielded considerable influence in the surgical societies. His personal wait and see attitude toward early open-heart surgery did not prevent him from publicly applauding Lillehei for his ingenuity and accomplishments. DeBakey, too, was an imaginative tinkerer, but he was still busy building Baylor and his burgeoning practice. The 202 open-heart surgeries Cooley had done with the DeWall-Lillehei oxygenator was more than twice what Lillehei and Kirklin had done combined, but DeBakey remained unconvinced.

In Minnesota, working with the engineers at Baxter Travenol in 1957, DeWall and Vincent Gott, another Lillehei team member, produced a commercially available version, and the DeWall-Lillehei oxygenator was there for the purchasing: ready to use, pre-sterilized, sealed in a plastic bag, disposable, and all at a price of about fifty dollars. This was unthinkable just five years after the calamities associated with the hugely expensive Dennis behemoth and the Gibbon machine. By contrast, even Kirklin's successful version represented an investment of more than fifty thousand dollars—in 1956—and required an enormous team to operate it.

A simple, affordable, fifty-dollar, heart-lung bypass machine was now available for heart surgeons everywhere. Its wide acceptance after Cooley's endorsement sowed the seeds for cardiac surgery in hospitals across the country. Cooley had already amassed, by far, the largest experience, and yet, for the next several years, virtually all the significant advances in survival rates would still come from Lillehei and Kirklin. Cooley, with his enormous practice and great surgical skill, was not wed to the lab and problem solving, as were the two who had preceded him.

★ ★ ★ ★ ★

As the number of open-heart cases increased, the number of deaths increased as well. Not surprisingly, some were due to the weakened state of the children, who tended to succumb to pneumonia which had taken Gregory Glidden's life when Lillehei first began. With experience, it became clear that children a year or two older did better than infants during surgery. A balance was sought between the effects of repeated lung disease and the benefits of waiting. But curiously, children who died in the immediate post-surgical period were not always the most critically ill.

It was also very significant that most of the deaths occurred in patients with issues that included VSDs. Most postoperative deaths were among those whose hearts could not be restarted or could not be returned to normal rhythm after coming off bypass. This was true with cross-circulation, and later, with every version of the heart-lung machines. Stopping hearts to facilitate surgery made it all possible, and at the completion of surgery, the patient's heartbeat had to be restored. It was the inability to restore normal heart rhythm that had resulted in altogether too many unexplained deaths.

In 1953, when ASD repairs were being done under hypothermia, there were tense moments waiting for a heartbeat to return. Watchful waiting during rewarming, and sometimes cardiac massage, were the rule. The same approach applied with cross-circulation, or whatever bypass was being employed. Restoring a normal rhythm after ASD repair was almost always successful.

When VSD surgery began a year later, the number of problems escalated. Some 20 percent of the young patients undergoing VSD repair developed what is termed complete heart block, a condition in which the pulse rate slows to fewer than forty beats per minute, too slow to sustain life for most patients.

Lillehei and Kirklin, the only surgeons in the world doing VSD repairs at the time, both noted the increased mortality, which was for no apparent reason. Their approach to the problem would graphically demonstrate the fundamental difference between the two men.

Kirklin scoured the literature and studied the electrical conduction system of the heart. Recently published work had indicated that specialized heart muscle, or myocardial cells, carried the message to beat from the sinoatrial node, located high on the septum between the atria, down to the atrioventricular node, located between the atrial septum and ventricular septum. In mechanical terms, these nodes could be thought of as junction boxes along an electrical pathway. The impulse from the atrioventricular node is then carried within the ventricular septum to another node called the bundle of His, (pronounced hiss) from which pacemaking impulses are divided into right and left bundles. Without continuity of this electrical pathway, the heartbeat would be slowed, interrupted, or stopped.

Most often, the location of the bundle of His coincides with the lowermost aspect of a VSD, and therefore, correcting either pure VSDs or tetralogy of Fallot defects, of which a VSD is an integral part, was fraught with danger. The bundle can be thought of as being imbedded in the septum on one side of the hole or the other. Simply suturing the VSD closed ran the risk of damaging the bundle and causing heart block.

Kirklin's approach was to avoid suturing where the bundle should be, though he could not actually see it. By moving suture placement in the lower aspect of the defect, Kirklin reduced mortality figures from 20 percent to less than 5 percent. Death from heart block went from one in five, to one in twenty, a dramatic, lifesaving advance.

Lillehei thought the bundle of His was a myth. And since he could not visualize it grossly or microscopically, he sought another solution when heart block occurred. His solution was not to prevent it, which he thought impossible, but to keep the heart beating with external electrical stimulation when heart block occurred.

The idea was not a new one. Physiologists had been stimulating frog hearts with electrical impulses for decades. Each impulse caused a contraction of the ventricle, and a heartbeat. In the early 1950s, Wilfred Bigelow, the father of hypothermia, noted that some of the dogs in his hypothermia experiments had developed heart blocks as their body temperatures were lowered. Bigelow solved the problem by pacing their hearts with external electrical impulses. The procedure had been successful, but once again, Bigelow was not the first to bring his experimental finding to human application. Another surgeon preempted him and took Bigelow's work from the lab to the operating room, and it didn't turn out to be as simple as expected.

The shocking procedure was exquisitely painful to patients. Each impulse was like the jolt of electrical paddles used in cardiac arrest, literally bouncing the patient off the bed. When this was continued with the patient awake, each heartbeat inducing shock was painful, and the procedure was quickly abandoned.

It is unclear whether Lillehei was aware of Bigelow's pacing experience in the dog lab, or the brief trial of human shocking. However, during a morbidity and mortality conference at University Hospital—a hospital meeting where untoward outcomes are discussed—the topic was the death of a tetralogy of Fallot patient from heart block. A physiologist from the medical school mentioned that he used low voltage pacing for frog hearts and it worked well. Lillehei assigned his resident, Vincent Gott, to look into the matter in the dog lab. Gott was the same young surgeon who had been instrumental in taking the DeWall-Lillehei heart-lung machine from bottles and tubes to commercial viability. He, and another resident, Mansur Taufic, found that they could induce complete heart block in a dog, insert a single wire from a low voltage stimulator into the heart, another on the skin for grounding, and successfully pace the dog's heart at whatever rate they wished by increasing or decreasing the frequency of the stimulating impulse, without inducing shocks.

Gott didn't rush to report his success to Lillehei, thinking that one couldn't simply stick an electrical wire into the heart of a human patient and leave it there. But he underestimated his mentor. When another resident mentioned their dog lab success to Lillehei, he responded to the information with a typical "Why not?" If a patient faced death from complete heart block, why not try low voltage electrical stimulation?

On January 30, 1957, another of Lillehei's patients developed heart block. A resident was quickly dispatched to bring the electrical stimulator from the dog lab to the operating room while the heart was massaged manually to keep the child alive. When the stimulator arrived, the wires were inserted into the boy's heart and to a grounding area, the machine was plugged into an electrical outlet, switched on, and instantly, the moribund heart began to beat. This was an historical first. No human heart rhythm had ever been comfortably produced by external stimulation before.

The idea was to stimulate the heart to beat until the electrical system of the heart took over. The gap between the need for external pacing and the restoration of normal heart rhythm varied from days to weeks, and in some cases, months. Still, it worked. Going forward, Lillehei prepared for this eventuality by implanting electrodes at the close of every surgery and bringing the insulated wires out through the skin. They would be in place if the need arose. When normal rhythm was restored, it rarely reverted to heart block, and the wires were easily dislodged and pulled out through the skin with no ill effects. Of course, the idea of wires attached to the heart being brought outside the body carried with it the fear of infection. It was a two way street. Lillehei thought that tunneling the wire under the skin for some distance would offer protection against infection. Decades of indwelling arterial and venous lines had proven well tolerated, so why not wires? It was a good guess, based on very little, but, as it turned out, there was no infection problem. Occasionally, in the longer-term cases, scar tissue developed around the wires, and increasingly higher voltages were required to maintain pacing. That worked as well. The only real hitch was that the patient was connected to an electrical socket and had to remain tethered by a long electrical cord until normal function returned.

Nine months later, on Halloween of 1957, a major power outage struck the Minneapolis area. As it happened, one of Lillehei's young post-operative patients with heart block was being paced when the power went down. With no adequate secondary power source in the hospital, the stimulator stopped pacing and the child died.

The tragedy convinced Lillehei that the pacemaker had to be self-contained, and battery powered. At the time, University Hospital intermittently employed an electrical instrument repairman named Earl Bakken, a tinkerer and self-described nerd. Bakken also owned a tiny electronics and television repair business with his brother-in-law. The company, with the serious sounding name, Medtronic. Inc., was housed in a family garage in northwest Minneapolis. The garage itself had been constructed from two double-wide trailers. It was jam packed with circuitry, meters, wiring, vacuum tubes, and deconstructed electronic gadgets, and could have been a mad scientist movie set.

Lillehei asked Bakken if he could make a self-contained, portable, battery-driven, low-voltage stimulator to replace the plug-in system that had just cost a life. Bakken agreed to try, and a month later delivered a device based on the diagram for a transistorized metronome he had seen in *Popular Electronics* magazine. Transistors had been invented at Bell Laboratories in 1947 and were all the rage among electronics hobbyists. In 1950, the first transistor radio was introduced, realizing the possibilities of miniaturization. The little radios were everywhere, changing the way music and news were consumed, and presaging a social phenomenon. For engineers, the transistor was about to lead to the world of printed circuits, microchips, and computers. Large devices powered by multiple vacuum tubes were rapidly being made obsolete by tiny, energy saving, transistorized circuits.

The transistorized stimulator Bakken produced was four and a half inches square, and an inch and a half thick. It was housed in a metal case with dials on the face for controlling heart rate, exactly as the metronome circuit adjusted time. Lillehei was delighted with the little box. It could be placed on a bedside table, easily moved around, and most importantly, it wasn't plugged into the wall.

Lillehei asked Bakken to deliver the device to the lab where Vincent Gott would implant it in a dog with surgically created heart block. If the pacing succeeded, the plan was to produce a more sophisticated version for human use. But when Bakken returned to the lab the next day, the device had vanished. Working late the previous night, Lillehei found a patient in trouble. He rushed to the lab, saw how well the portable pacemaker was functioning, disconnected it from the dog, brought it to the hospital, and immediately connected it to a post-operative child suffering complete heart block. In April of 1958, the first battery operated, portable pacemaker was born.

From then on, pacemaker technology moved at lightning speed. Smaller versions capable of being strapped to the patient followed, allowing freedom and mobility. Soon, fully implantable pacemakers powered by mercury batteries became available, which were soon supplanted by long-life lithium batteries. Today's ubiquitous pacemakers barely resemble the crude contraption Bakken created to Lillehei's design, and more than a million of the lifesaving devices are installed worldwide every year. Medtronic Inc., Bakken's little garage-based shop, is currently the world's largest medical device company, doing some $31 billion in annual sales.

The existential questions remained: whose solution to the problem of heart block was more appropriate, which saved more lives, and which did more for medicine and mankind? The answers were quite obvious and defined the very nature of the two men.

Kirklin was a man of pure, hard facts and actuarial tables, while Lillehei was a man of action and practical solutions. Both were men of science and both trained a widely-branched tree of distinguished cardiac surgeons. Kirklin's legacy was the Mayo-Gibbon heart-lung bypass machine, which he scrupulously perfected and made available to the world. And operating in his linear manner, he made his protocols for bundle of His and heart block a standard technique.

Lillehei, on the other hand, approached the problem in a less anatomic, if not less scientific manner. But his solution gave birth to the entire pacemaker industry and has saved millions of lives for nearly seven decades.

Despite their frequently divergent approaches, the two remained friendly throughout their careers, and never spoke harshly of one another.

★ ★ ★ ★ ★

Through the late 1950s, Lillehei and the work forged in Minnesota were no longer a local secret, and even the old school surgeons no longer denied his role in pioneering and advancing open-heart surgery. By 1960, one thousand open-heart sur-geries, many of them innovative breakthroughs; an affordable, workable, bypass machine; and a battery-powered pacemaker had cemented Lillehei's position as the leader of cardiac surgery innovation.

Surgeons from around the world flocked to Minneapolis and Lillehei became a widely coveted lecturer, frequently cov-ered by the media. Perhaps more importantly, in the arc of the discipline, the talented young men who would move open-heart surgery to heights only imagined by Lillehei himself, were among those who came to train with him. Best known among them were Christiaan Barnard and Norman Shumway. The former would become internationally famous for per-forming the world's first successful heart transplant, the latter the undisputed father of the procedure. Both were risk tak-ers on a well-lit stage. Their stories would soon consume the world, while numerous others quietly became leaders of heart surgery around the world.

Though Minneapolis served as the birthplace of open-heart surgery, Houston was about to become its epicenter. There, Michael Ellis DeBakey and Denton Arthur Cooley would perform staggering numbers of surgeries, repeatedly garner covers of *Time* and *Life*, become household names, and principals in the most infamous feud in medical history. And if the risks taken by Lillehei generated heated ethical quandaries, that was just the beginning. Legal issues were about to bleed into prosecutions, felony convictions, social disgrace, and aca-demic ignominy.

CHAPTER TWELVE

HOUSTON

When Denton Cooley rose to defend Walt Lillehei and the DeWall-Lillehei bypass machine, he had been a relatively unknown thirty-six-year-old Texan. His statement about the efficacy of the machine shocked the entire audience that hadn't a combined open-heart surgery experience nearly as great as his 202 cases. He simply stopped the proceedings cold. If his sole purpose was to shut down Lillehei's detractors, it also immediately placed Cooley at the forefront of cardiac surgery.

Cooley was only two years younger than Lillehei and their early lives were quite similar. Both were the sons of dentists, with families prominent in their communities. The Lillehei's were firmly entrenched in Minneapolis. The Cooley roots in Houston were as deep and even more profound. From the arrival of his paternal grandfather as a real estate developer in 1891, the Cooley's prospered with the oil boom that fed the growth of the city. Cooley's father, like Lillehei's, had material success, and neither boy wanted for anything. Both described some of the happiest moments of their boyhoods acquiring and rebuilding Model T Fords and the misadventures it spawned. Both were self-described as shy and both were schooled near home, Lillehei at the University of Minnesota, and Cooley at the University of Texas in Austin. Both were unusually handsome young men driven by ambition and both were honor students throughout their school careers. If Lillehei's gifts were imagination and dogged pursuit, Cooley's were technical genius and the ability to maximize what others had envisioned. With personalities and gifts markedly divergent, they recognized in one another a great vision for cardiac surgery and respect for the unusual qualities the other brought to the table.

In college, Cooley, at six-foot-four, was a varsity basketball star, a very good tennis player, and an avid golfer. In addition to an obsession with sports, Cooley had an active fraternity life. As one of the select few to be invited to join the "Cowboys," he was literally branded with the UT symbol of the University of Texas. It was real branding, Texas style, with a white-hot iron. As Cooley tells it, in the first pass, the iron wasn't hot enough to complete the job and he had it reheated and reapplied to his skin. For the rest of his life, he proudly exposed the longhorn brand on his chest whenever the opportunity arose. Quietly fun loving, Cooley was an academic star as well. His confidence grew with success, and he became outgoing, graceful, and socially adept. Entering medical school at the beginning of the war, he spent two years at the top of his class at the University of Texas Medical Branch, in Galveston, and then, heeding some good advice, used his excellent record to transfer to Johns Hopkins University Medical School, one of the premier institutions in the country.

Cooley, from the University of Texas Medical Branch, entered Johns Hopkins uneasy about competing with students from the elite eastern colleges. That fear abated quickly. He did exceedingly well from the start and found it far from a grind. Skipping a surgical clinic to play tennis on his first fine spring day in Baltimore, he was chagrinned to find himself observed by Dr. Alfred Blalock, the new chief of surgery, who had been strolling by the courts on his way from the clinic Cooley had skipped. Instead of calling him out for missing clinic, Blalock motioned him over and said, "I've been watching your tennis game. You're a pretty good player." Cooley, who envisioned his Hopkins career going out the window, was much relieved. From that point on, a mentorship, and then a friendship, developed. Blalock was a southern gentleman, rarely seen without a cigarette in a long black holder and a big smile. The two bonded, and Blalock and Cooley enjoyed evenings of ping pong and whiskey, two pastimes at which Cooley excelled. He spent a good deal of time with the Blalock family, and from his mentor, felt the strong pull toward a career in surgery.

Cooley began his internship at Hopkins in 1944, and when Blalock performed the first "blue baby" operation, he was a junior member of the team. Not only was Blalock's success a watershed moment in surgery, but the worldwide fame it brought the surgeon had not been lost on Cooley.

The success of the Taussig-Blalock operation, and the enormous publicity surrounding it, filled the wards. Hundreds of children afflicted with the tetralogy of Fallot were brought from Taussig at the Children's Heart Clinic to Blalock's surgical service. Soon, the "blue babies" consumed Blalock's time. The prominence that had won him his chair at Hopkins was based on his work treating shock and replacing blood volume, crucial advances in wartime, but not actual surgery. It must have come as something of a surprise for a man known primarily as a research surgeon, and never fully confident in the operating room, to have found himself in such an exalted position. Blalock was not a great operating surgeon, but his intellect, genial manner, and gift for inspiration produced a generation of surgical leaders.

After completing his internship, Cooley was surprised to have been asked to become Blalock's cardiac resident, an unusual promotion for a neophyte surgeon. But Cooley had shown enormous skill and dexterity and was delighted with the offer. He took to it with ease and was soon performing the Taussig-Blalock operation himself, having never done so much as simple gall bladder surgery. The experience convinced him that he would become a cardiovascular surgeon.

In 1946, Cooley, junior surgical resident at Johns Hopkins, became First Lieutenant Denton Cooley. Blalock offered to help get Cooley assigned to Walter Reed Hospital so that he would have a wide surgical experience and continue to be in contact with nearby Johns Hopkins.

With that attempt to influence his assignment, Cooley had the first of a lifetime of clashes with Michael DeBakey. Dispatched to the Surgeon General's office in Washington with his letter from Blalock, Cooley never got past the Surgeon General's adjutant—one Michael DeBakey. The request, if it had ever reached the general, was ignored, and Cooley was promptly sent off to spend two years as a surgeon in Germany and Austria.

Far from the ivory tower of Johns Hopkins, the assignment proved pleasant and profitable. There, sports took top priority yet again. Cooley even used a phony excuse to beg out of joining a teaching tour Blalock was making in London and Paris, in order to compete in a tennis tournament. His European surgical experience was primarily emergency surgery resulting from civilian injuries and illness. The war was over and serious surgical patients were airlifted to larger, better equipped hospitals. Cooley did not miss the lack of challenge and made up for it with travel, tennis, basketball, and partying.

Returning as chief resident, he was assigned to the cardiovascular service. Johns Hopkins was structured in the Halsted system of increasing responsibility and he had total autonomy in dealing with his patients. There, he had his initial experience excising sac-like aortic aneurysms, the procedure that would surprise DeBakey when he began working for him at Baylor.

Cooley was happy back at Hopkins, and as was his style, he worked and played hard. Popular with the nurses for his good looks and amusing manner, he was liked by his co-residents for his social ease, athletic ability, and was respected for his superior technical skill and dexterity by the senior staff. It was an easy journey and as free of potholes as all of Cooley's journeys had been.

During that chief resident year, Cooley met and married Louise Thomas, the pretty head nurse on the Halsted surgical ward. The following year, they had the first of their five daughters. Planning to return home to Houston to practice, Cooley secured a position at Baylor, the only academic surgical service in town, which was now led by the same straight arrow— DeBakey—whom he suspected of depositing his letter to the Surgeon General in the circular file.

Lord Russell Brock, then still Mr. Brock, a pioneering British cardiovascular surgeon, had been visiting professor at Hopkins for a month during Cooley's chief resident year. Stiff collared, slick haired, immaculately dressed, sporting round spectacles, and as tight as a rolled umbrella, Brock appeared the least likely candidate to be a risk taker. And yet, he was one of the first to perform blind, intracardiac fracture of calcified valves, along with his cultural opposite, the adventurous, outspoken American, Charles Bailey. Brock was impressed by Cooley's skill and demeanor and invited him to spend a year as his assistant. It was a unique opportunity, and he and Louise were excited about living in London. Without too much difficulty, Cooley convinced DeBakey to hold his slot at Baylor for a year.

It was not a taxing year, part post graduate education, part boondoggle. The Cooley's traveled extensively, hosted visiting family and friends, and with their young daughter, Mary, had their first opportunity to spend time together as a family. On the training front, before the year was out, Cooley was bored with time spent in diagnostic and experimental labs, calling Brock's intensive patient study "Sherlock Holmes style." He wanted to operate and he wanted to get back to Houston. Brock, who was aware of Cooley's restlessness, commented sometime later, "He believed he had gotten as much in nine months here as the average man would have gotten in a year— probably true. It stands to reason that the world will not produce another Denton Cooley: and, frankly, I have my doubts if the world could handle another one. He spun in and out of here like a whirlwind, though not without leaving his mark— indeed, several marks."

In June of 1951, Cooley, the now pregnant Louise, and young Mary arrived in Houston to begin their new lives. Cooley was happy to be in his hometown and excited to begin the career he had been training for. The Texas Medical Center was still comprised of only Jefferson Davis, the charity hospital, the Hermann Hospital, the VA Hospital, and Baylor University college of Medicine. The new Methodist Hospital, the jewel in the crown, would open the following year.

Cooley's extraordinary performance excising an aneurysm on his first workday was a signal to DeBakey that he had found the right young man to help him grow the vascular surgery practice. DeBakey's revolutionary Dacron graft landed him, and to a lesser extent, his junior partner, on center stage as the process came of age. Through 1955, DeBakey and Cooley performed more than two hundred and fifty aortic graft surgeries, and out of nowhere, Houston had become the aneurysm center of the world.

The next target was the carotid artery, the major vessel supplying blood to the brain. Atherosclerosis, the disease that occludes arteries, can do critical damage to the carotid artery. Reduced blood supply causes reduced oxygen supply, and everything from mental impairment to stroke and death can result. In 1956, Cooley performed the world's first successful operation to clear the plaques from the carotid artery, a procedure called an endarterectomy. It was risky business. The procedure required clamping off the blood supply to the brain while the artery was opened and reamed clean, and the possibility of dislodging a plaque and causing a stroke was real. To minimize the possibility of brain damage from anoxia, Cooley devised a localized version of hypothermia to reduce brain metabolism and reduce oxygen requirements. The system was as crude and simple as placing the patient's head into a bucket of ice, which is exactly what he did. He also rigged a minor shunt with large bore needles and tubing in an attempt to divert some oxygenated blood around the clamped off area and allow at least a trickle to circulate to the brain.

It was an untested premise, and the first case suffered shaky moments. After a few hours of postoperative weakness and partial paralysis, the patient fully recovered and a new lifesaving procedure was born. From that point on, the team performed the operation frequently and reported it widely. DeBakey, with Cooley as his assistant, had attempted the same procedure several months previously, but he had aborted the operation when the blockage couldn't be cleared. Despite his own obvious failure, DeBakey promoted the procedure as his invention, and regularly spoke of having performed the first successful carotid endarterectomy. Cooley fumed. It was a classic example of selective memory which Cooley never forgot.

Over the next two years, separately, and together, they performed more than seventy-five carotid endarterectomies. Soon after their first report, the operation became a routine tool in the vascular surgeon's kit. In addition to hundreds of aneurysm grafts and carotid endarterectomies, both Cooley and DeBakey were also doing blind mitral and aortic valvulotomies in the manner of Bailey and Brock. It was 1955, and they still were not doing open-heart surgery.

In February of that year, the Society of University Surgeons met in Houston. DeBakey and Cooley were a constant presence in the host city. A much-anticipated event at the meeting was Lillehei's movie of his cross-circulation procedure. The movie was as dramatic as had been expected, and the radical concept received a mixed reception. But Lillehei had already done dozens of cases, and his success in saving previously unsalvageable young lives couldn't be denied. DeBakey was among the first to stand and offer his compliments, but neither he nor virtually anyone else in the audience was prepared to follow Lillehei over the precipice.

At few months later, at a meeting in the spring of 1955, Kirklin reported having used his modified Gibbon machine on eight cases at the Mayo Clinic with four survivors. When Cooley cornered DeBakey and claimed that they could build the same sort of machine cheaper, he was met with more than financial resistance. DeBakey told his junior partner that he had already assigned two staff members to the bypass machine project, and Cooley's input wasn't necessary. Cooley was stung. In addition to claiming Cooley's firsts as his own, DeBakey was now excluding him from what he knew was the future.

DeBakey filled the departmental purse through government grants and local donations and held the purse strings tightly. He made no attempt to disguise the fact that he would in no way support Cooley's acquisition of a bypass machine, nor would his young associate be included in his own plans to develop one. After a scant four years at Baylor, Cooley was perceived as a looming threat to the supremacy of Michael DeBakey.

Cooley knew the DeWall-Lillehei machine was the answer. No longer confiding in DeBakey, nor even asking his permission, Cooley and two medical students constructed a DeWall-Lillehei machine. Through the winter and early spring of 1956, Cooley's team experimented with his new machine in the dog lab. But although the machine supported the surgery properly, the dogs ultimately hemorrhaged and died. It was a frustrating learning curve. He knew the problem was unique to canine surgery and that it didn't translate directly to humans, but he had to succeed before daring to introduce the machine into the operating room.

Then, on April 5, 1956, he received an urgent call from a cardiologist caring for a patient at another hospital who had suffered a cataclysmic myocardial infarct.The severely compromised coronary blood flow had led to the loss of much of the septum between his ventricles. The cardiologist, aware of the abysmal results of the work in the dog lab, made it clear that unless the huge hole in the patient's ventricular septum was repaired immediately, he would be dead before the day was out. Any chance was better than none. Cooley didn't press about his lack of success in the dog lab. He saw his opportunity and took it.The moribund patient was transferred to Methodist. Cooley believed that the machine worked for Lillehei, and it would work for him. In any case, the emergency situation changed the rules.This was a rationale that Cooley would employ again and would nearly lead to his undoing.

And so, the stage was set for Cooley's debut open-heart surgery. If he did not operate, the patient would certainly die. If he did operate, the massive tissue loss might be irreparable, and the patient would die. If the machine failed, the patient would die. But, if the stars aligned, Cooley might save the patient, and he would be a hero. He would also have the first operational bypass machine at Methodist Hospital, the first in Texas, and the first outside of Minnesota. Denton Cooley would be an open-heart surgeon to be reckoned with.

With only twenty-five minutes on bypass, Cooley reconstructed the septum with a synthetic patch of Ivalon sponge and the patient survived. Both the bypass machine and the introduction of foreign substances for heart repair came courtesy of Lillehei. But this was Texas, not Minnesota, and Cooley was now a local celebrity. He had his machine in the operating room and his foot in the door. In rapid succession, he did six more cases using the DeWall-Lillehei pump. All survived and left the hospital. Six weeks after surgery, the groundbreaking first patient died of multiple complications. But having gotten seven patients on the pump, their defects corrected, and off the pump, Cooley proved his point. By the time the year was out, he'd performed one hundred open-heart operations and was the busiest heart surgeon in the world.

All of this did not sit well with DeBakey. The idea that his junior associate was the man of the hour drove the wedge deeper between them. As Cooley began doing large numbers of open-heart cases, he soon found it difficult to come by enough disposable sterile tubing for the pump. With that minor procurement problem, and perhaps because he wanted a machine of his own, Cooley, and two associates, developed their own pump oxygenator closely based on the DeWall-Lillehei device. It was made of stainless steel, easily sterilized, and didn't require the hard to come by disposable tubing. The slightly sleeker device looked like a percolator and was nicknamed "Cooley's Coffeepot." The machine was financed by private donations and small grants secured by Cooley. No department funds or federal grants had been used, nor had permission to proceed been sought from DeBakey.

Unwilling to sit by as his junior star rose, DeBakey scheduled a VSD repair, which he had never attempted before. Without speaking to Cooley, he appropriated the Coffeepot for the case. Cooley got wind of it and was outraged. He drove to DeBakey's home, and for the first time, faced off against his boss. DeBakey made the erroneous case that his department had funded the machine and therefore it was Baylor property. Cooley did not back down, DeBakey blinked, and eventually the case was moved to Texas Children's Hospital and done by

Cooley. It was just another minor skirmish within the insular Baylor community, but the two men were now barely speaking.

Despite dramatic surgeries like Cooley's first pump patient who had been an adult, children with congenital heart defects continued to comprise the majority of open-heart cases, and they were now flocking to Houston in great numbers. After performing some two hundred and fifty operations with the Coffeepot, Cooley abandoned it in favor of the new commercial version of the DeWall-Lillehei machine, which was being produced and sold by the Baxter Travenol company. Maintaining the same concept, the new device was even simpler, contained in a plastic pouch and entirely disposable. His surgical technique minimized pump time, boasting an average of seven minutes on pump to repair an ASD, which, though it seems miraculously fast, was exactly John Lewis's open-heart time for his first ASD under hypothermia.

Pump time has a linear relationship to survival and an inverse relationship to complications. The less time on the pump the better. Cooley was fast and he wanted to be faster. His results were excellent and he wanted them to be better. As disposable pumps made preparation easier and his waiting list grew, he rethought the whole process to identify the bottle neck that prevented him from doing more surgery.

Circulation through the heart, arteries, veins, and back to the heart is a closed system that carries oxygen bound to red blood cells, but not free oxygen. Free oxygen, or air bubbles, are catastrophic. In all open-heart surgery, survival is dependent on preventing air bubbles, or air emboli, from reaching the brain. To prevent this from happening, the pump, the reservoir, and all tubing are filled with blood, maintaining a closed, air free, system. At the end of the operation, the chambers of the heart, which had been excluded from circulation and intentionally kept virtually blood free for visibility, are filled to the point of overflowing with blood, purging the free air before the incision in the heart is closed. The need for maintaining the closed system has been known from the beginning of the adventure of heart surgery. Breeches in continuity resulted in death in Clarence Dennis's second attempt in 1951, and in permanent brain damage for the mother of one of Lillehei's cross-circulation patients. In both instances, an anesthesiologist accidently introduced air through a vein. But not purging air from a surgically opened heart was the direct cause of death in Bailey's attempt to do the first ASD repair. The lesson hard learned by loss of lives was to keep the closed system air free.

Using the pump required eight to ten units of fresh, type-matched blood available on the morning of surgery. That included the five units of blood necessary to fill the reservoir, the pump, and the tubing. This process is called priming the pump. Every sort of mechanical pump is primed to create a closed system which allows it to function smoothly. But collecting matched blood prior to surgery was a daunting, time-consuming task. It overtaxed the blood banks and made doing more than a single operation in a day extremely difficult. With inexpensive pumps, pump time of less than half an hour, and total operating time of under an hour, priming the pump was the bottle neck preventing Cooley from doing more surgery.

Cooley had the pump, the patients, the skill, and a simple solution that revolutionized open-heart surgery. He primed the pump with an IV solution of dextrose and distilled water instead of blood. Others had tried the solution as well, but Cooley moved an experimental concept to an operative routine. Not needing to collect large volumes of fresh blood relieved the mounting pressure that open-heart surgery was putting on already strained blood banks.

Cooley could now schedule multiple operations each day. With his skilled staff preparing, opening, and closing, he could appear for the actual cardiac repair and move to the next operation on the production line. He was soon performing more heart surgery in a week than many centers were doing in a year. By the end of 1962, his method of priming the pump with dextrose in water had generally supplanted the use of blood priming, and he had already used the technique on 241 patients without incident. With the availability of efficient, inexpensive, disposable bypass machines, heart surgery was generally available around the country. Priming the pump with water made it easier, faster, and more efficient.

Cooley was on top of the world. But with his success, the fracture with DeBakey was no longer a secret. The two had been working physically apart since 1954, when Texas Children's hospital and St. Luke's opened. Cooley was operating primarily at St. Luke's and Texas Children's, where four floors had been devoted to accommodating his needs. He had his own operating rooms, his own patient floors, and even moved his offices to the new facility. Although he was the least research oriented of the cardiac cowboys, he had his own research labs.

The new hospitals were only a few hundred yards from Methodist, Baylor, and DeBakey. The two surgeons were still associated academically and financially but had as little to do with one another as possible. The atmosphere became generally uncomfortable for everyone around them. The Cooley's still lived on Cherokee Street, near the DeBakey's. The families were initially close, but three years later, they socialized only at hospital related events. The resident staff worked closely with both surgeons, and it was impossible to be unaware of the frost that had settled on the relationship.

Largely, this was because Cooley felt unwelcome and unappreciated. He had been excluded from the plans for the Baylor heart-lung machine, which never quite materialized. His credit for his aneurysm work and carotid endarterectomy had been co-opted and he had generally been disregarded at a time when he had already become the biggest producer at the Texas Medical Center.

The DeBakey camp never discussed the cause for the rift, but it was generally believed that the boss felt his supremacy and authority were challenged. But it didn't take a challenge for DeBakey to lash out. Habitually demeaning and cruel to his underlings, he often banished residents from the program for minor transgressions, true or imagined. Challenge had not been necessary for this side of his nature to surface.

DeBakey was an innovator, researcher, teacher, fundraiser, empire builder, and a world class publicity seeker. As a surgeon, he was doubtlessly accomplished, and he stood out among others, until Cooley arrived. Cooley was unique. He wasn't merely accomplished, he was a savant among surgeons. Every move was efficient. He was fast without seeming to rush, and he was able to make difficult maneuvers look easy, instinctively able to visualize the best way to proceed. These attributes alone could be expected to draw resident staff to him. But he was also unfailingly polite to all levels of staff, both in the operating room, and out. The young doctors were awe struck by his work, and felt as comfortable and honored to be around Cooley as they felt fearful around DeBakey.

Cooley had been surprised upon first witnessing DeBakey's behavior in the operating room. To a lesser degree, he had seen similar behavior at Hopkins. The revered Alfred Blalock was prone to bursts of anger at surgery, almost always followed by an apology. And he was, at all other times, a warm human being, gracious and beloved by students and peers alike. Those around Blalock attributed his outbursts to insecurity during surgery, for whatever else he had accomplished, he was not comfortable operating.

Initially, Cooley thought he was witnessing more of the same. But DeBakey was too good a surgeon to be unsure of himself. And, in fact, his demeaning outbursts were not confined to the operating room. The same explosive temper would surface unexpectedly during rounds, meetings, and sometimes in simple conversation. Cooley found it both hard to understand and hard to forgive. How could this same man be saint-like toward his patients, well-mannered and gentlemanly among his fellow administrators, government officials, and benefactors, and a horror elsewhere? Once the pattern became clear, it was another lever in the schism between them.

★　★　★　★　★

As the decade turned to the 1960s, forty-year-old Cooley was the father of five daughters and living well. He had convinced DeBakey to alter their financial deal with Baylor, serving both handsomely by allowing them to keep a larger percentage of their billings. It had been an exceptional eight years.

Cooley was doing four times as many cases as DeBakey and was building a loyal staff around him. He was happier working at Children's and St. Luke's, and every day seemed to brighten his star. The weekends were for family, tennis, and golf, and the Cooley's managed to socialize often. Work hours were work hours. They began early and ended late, but they didn't come home with him. From the very beginning, he had been cool and detached. When he worked, he worked relentlessly, and it had all been very easy. He had good looks, social ease, uncanny surgical skill, ambition, and the ego to go along with it. For Cooley, the 1960s would be a decade of great personal achievements, prosperity, and fame, ending in infamy.

★   ★   ★   ★   ★

John Gibbon began the search for a heart-lung bypass machine after standing by helplessly while a young woman died from massive pulmonary emboli. These blood clots usually originate in veins of the legs or abdomen, propagate in the great veins and move through the pulmonary circulation, lodge in the lungs, prevent oxygenation of blood, and essentially suffocate the victim.

In 1962, Cooley used the heart-lung bypass machine to facilitate removal of pulmonary emboli from the lungs of a moribund patient, bringing full circle the quest begun by Gibbon thirty years earlier. The heroic operation required only fifteen minutes of pump time. The procedure was a first, which made it notable in the history of the heart-lung bypass machine, but its real importance was in the routine leading up to the surgery. Swift action such as this had been made possible by the simplicity of priming the pump with glucose and water instead of having to wait for liters of matched blood to become available. It was a Cooley simplification with enormous impact on the practice of cardiac surgery. It wasn't named or patented; it just changed the way open-heart surgery was done.

The 1960s were a period of head spinning advances in a field that hadn't existed a decade before. In 1962, the Starr-Edwards artificial aortic valve became commercially available. What might appear an asterisk in the history of cardiac surgery was actually the first page in a catalogue of replacement parts.

The aortic valve separates the left ventricle from the aorta. In nature, it is made of three separate leaves, and in the open position, they allow oxygenated blood under pressure to be pumped out of the left ventricle into the aorta. This is the phase called systole. In the closed position, it prevents back-flow of blood from the aorta into the left ventricle during relaxation, or diastole. The leaflets of the valve are opened and closed by the pressure gradients between ventricle and aorta. When disease affects the aortic valve, the leaflets can be frozen in a nearly closed position called stenosis. This aortic stenosis impedes the flow of oxygenated blood from the heart to the vital organs, Conversely, the valve might become frozen open and unable to close completely. This condition is called incompetence, which allows regurgitation, or backflow of blood from the aorta. Though both of these conditions vary in degree, both can significantly interfere with normal heart function.

For twenty years, various surgical strategies were tried on heart valves following the blind approach to frozen mitral valves by Bailey and Brock. Most of the early work concentrated on the easily accessible mitral valve, the one most often targeted by rheumatic fever.

Replacing irreparable heart valves was a wholly new pursuit, unimaginable before the advent of the heart-lung bypass machine. Dwight Harken, who broke the heart surgery barrier by removing shrapnel fragments from within the heart, was the first to succeed at valve replacement as well. In 1960, he crafted and successfully implanted an aortic valve made of a cage and a silicone ball to mimic the action of the leaflets. Harken remained an active player in the evolution of cardiac surgery. His valve was functional, but his most significant contribution may have been devising the intensive care unit in 1951. First initiated for post cardiac surgery care patients, it quickly became the ICU, a ubiquitous component of critical patient care.

Barely a year after Harken's valve, Surgeon Albert Starr and engineer Lowell Edwards developed a similar device. Their valve employed a Lucite cage and a Silastic (vulcanized silicone rubber) ball. The Starr-Edwards valve became the first commercially available artificial heart valve, and with variations and improvements by people like Cooley and Lillehei, it remained a mainstay for aortic and mitral valve replacement for decades. Part of the beauty of the Starr-Edwards valve was its design. It was simply a silicone ball in a cage that opened and closed with the change in pressure between systole and diastole. It opened and allowed flow when the left ventricle contracted in systole, and closed to prevent backflow, or reflux, from the aorta when the ventricle relaxed and refilled during diastole, just like the natural aortic valve.

First onto the bandwagon was Cooley, with a reputation for taking on the most difficult cases and newest procedures. By the end of 1962, he had performed 111 aortic valve replacements with a constantly diminishing mortality rate, and more desperate patients flocked to his door.

By that time, the balance of power in Texas was shifting. DeBakey was still the department chair at Baylor, the surgeon in chief at Methodist, and the most famous vascular surgeon in the world. While open-heart surgery had captured his interest, his devotion was not nearly as singular as Cooley's. DeBakey's surgical load was enormous as well, he also wore more hats than his rival. Without referring to Cooley, DeBakey assembled a heart surgery team dedicated to his practice. But the facilities at Methodist were limited and open-heart surgery was already gravitating to the St. Luke's Texas Children's complex and Cooley. While DeBakey continued to run his empire at Methodist and Baylor, Cooley operated.

Without a lofty title or significant public exposure, Cooley's technical skill was celebrated across the medical community and his patient population grew to the edge of manageable proportions.

In less than ten years, open-heart surgery had become routine, and both Cooley and DeBakey sought larger stages. Cooley outgrew the four floors allotted to him at St. Luke's Episcopal and Texas Children's shortly after moving in. The echo of Cooley's success and the realization that open-heart surgery was taking wing around him inspired DeBakey to build a new, larger cardiovascular unit at Methodist, which plainly excluded Cooley. Cooley had his own plans. He established the Denton A. Cooley Foundation, and, in a stroke of genius, branded a nonprofit whose name told the story of where he was going. The new project was christened the Texas Heart Institute, logo signage and all. Cooley engaged lawyers and architects and proceeded on the premise that he could raise the funding for the THI solo. Ultimately, this proved naïve, and the boards of St Luke's and Texas Children's agreed that the THI should be incorporated into their planned expansion—a new, twenty-eight story complex composed of the two inpatient hospitals and Cooley's THI. Each would benefit from the presence of the others and the boards would meet together. Cooley alone donated $10 million of the projected $50 million needed for the complex.

The project was signed and sealed when DeBakey became aware of the scope of it. All this happened at his medical center, within his university, and the charge was being led by his junior partner—without him.

From fundraising to the 1967 groundbreaking, the reality of The Texas Heart Institute took five years.

However, on December 3, 1967, a shocking event stole the surgical limelight enjoyed by Cooley and DeBakey. It captured the attention of the world as no surgical feat ever had. On that day, an unknown, South African surgeon named Christiaan Barnard successfully transplanted a human heart, and overnight, became the most famous person in the world.

CHAPTER THIRTEEN

BARNARD

C hristiaan Neethling Barnard was charming, but not easy to like.

Nothing had been given to Barnard. He earned, or took, everything he achieved. Some might say he took what others earned. None can doubt that he saw the brass ring, grabbed it, and for better or worse, held it dear and lived a celebrated life of worldwide fame.

★ ★ ★ ★ ★

Of the four surgeons poised to perform the first heart transplant, Barnard was considered the least prepared. Groote Schuur Hospital sits at the picturesque base of Devil's Peak, near the Southern Atlantic. A teaching hospital affiliated with the University of Cape Town, Groote Schuur was unknown outside of South Africa prior to December 3, 1967. On that day, Barnard performed the first successful human to human heart transplant. The patient, Louis Washkansky, a grocer with end stage heart disease, lived eighteen days with the heart of twenty-five-year-old Denise Darvall beating in his fifty-three-year-old chest.

Barnard made history in his homeland of South Africa, but his history in heart surgery had begun, much like heart surgery itself, at the University of Minnesota, about as far from South Africa as one can travel.

Barnard was the third of four sons of a Dutch reformed minister in the hardscrabble wilderness of Cape Province. Vocally opposed to the repressive apartheid regime, his father served a poor church with a mixed-race population and was generally shunned by the controlling white population. Funds were always short, luxuries were absent, and education and self-sufficiency took their place. The children were encouraged not merely to succeed, but to be the best. The competitive and athletic Barnard ran a mile in record time in only his bare feet, won a tennis tournament with a borrowed racquet, and always did well in school. Despite the absence of the traditional trinkets of middle class life, it was not a deprived childhood. A strict mother and a principled father set the tone, and the few extras the family enjoyed were a small, very basic seaside vacation cottage, and a serviceable, old automobile.

Through frugality and a multitude of jobs, Reverend Barnard funded his children's educations. Christiaan attended medical school at the University of Cape Town, and in 1946, began his career as a rural family doctor. He quickly became bored with the general practice of medicine and returned to university as a surgical resident at Groote Schuur. There, Barnard developed an interest in intestinal surgery, doing laboratory research on intestinal atresia, a frequently lethal, embryological defect in which the intestine doesn't fully develop.

His work identified the vascular root of the problem and led to a lifesaving operation. Naturally, his stock rose quickly in the medical community. When he was offered the opportunity for further study under Owen Wangensteen at the University of Minnesota, Barnard leapt at the chance. It was December of 1955, Wangensteen was a world-renowned gastrointestinal surgeon and researcher, and it was a unique and unforeseen opportunity. With little money, a bare bones wardrobe, and great enthusiasm, Barnard happily traveled 8,817 miles to learn clinical surgery under Wangensteen.

Upon arriving in Minneapolis, his first unpleasant surprise was the punishing cold of the Minnesota winter. The second was being assigned to the Chief's laboratory projects rather than the clinical service.

Vincent Gott, one of Lillehei's fellows, was in charge of the heart surgery laboratory just across the hall from Wangensteen's lab. The researchers enjoyed an open door policy. Laboratory work included lots of watching and waiting, visiting, and bull sessions, which were routine among the young scientists. This was early in the era of the DeWall-Lillehei bubble oxygenator, and Barnard was fascinated by the experiments going on next door. Gott was working on aortic valve surgery, and Barnard quickly understood the problems and contributed to the wide-ranging discussions. Short staffed at surgery one day, Gott enlisted Barnard to operate the bypass machine. That was all it took. Three months after arriving in Minneapolis, he cajoled Wangensteen into allowing him to transfer to Lillehei's cardiac surgery service.

Initially, Barnard's wife, Aletta Gertruida Louw, Louwtjie to everyone, remained in Cape Town with their two children. Barnard found time to work hard on the Lillehei team, on his own projects for his PhD on intestinal atresia, as well as on his master of surgery thesis in aortic valve surgery. He also quickly found female company, and continued a lifelong, life wrecking pursuit of beautiful young women. His boyish good looks and confident, outgoing, personality were a winning combination in social situations, but not at all appreciated among his work colleagues. Most found him arrogant, self-centered, and self-promoting, a sore thumb among a team of relatively self-effacing Midwesterners.

Barnard spent two and a half years at the University of Minnesota and became part of Lillehei's crew. His seniors, Lillehei and Wangensteen, recognized his intellect, imagination, and work ethic. His colleagues were less receptive to his charm and outspoken, unconventional ideas. What Lillehei and Wangensteen liked, Barnard's coworkers saw as arrogant narcissism. Among those in whom Barnard engendered strong distaste was a slightly senior budding heart surgeon, Norman Shumway.

The off-putting acquaintanceship with Barnard would dog Shumway through a lifetime devoted to perfecting heart transplantation. It was Shumway who was primarily responsible for developing and refining the technique of heart transplantation, and he who had continued performing and refining the operation when others were despairing over the inability to conquer rejection. It was Shumway who had performed three hundred and fifty heart transplants in animals before having performed it clinically. It was Shumway who performed the first successful heart transplant in America, some weeks after Barnard's breakthrough. And, ultimately, it was Shumway who had quipped, "nobody remembers the second man to reach the North Pole."

Most of Barnard's time in Minnesota had been devoted to work. In addition to his hospital and laboratory duties, he had conjured up a grab bag of odd jobs to sustain him financially, save money to send for his family, and purchase a car. When, after six months, Louwitjie, and the children, Diedre and Andre joined him, Barnard continued his intense work schedule as well as his after-hours activities. The family spent a year in Minneapolis. The children had adapted happily and were becoming very American. But Louwitjie sensed the reasons for the virtual absence of her husband and decided it was best to return to Cape Town with the children.

In two and a half years at the University of Minnesota, Barnard completed the surgery, thoracic surgery, and cardiovascular surgery programs, and earned both his master's and PhD degrees. The success at multiple, simultaneous programs was Wangensteen-style total immersion, and Barnard's diligence and intelligence could not be doubted. He earned the respect of a unique coterie of superstars in the new field, including Lillehei, Varco, and Gott, but made few friends. Barnard alienated his wife and ran through a series of girlfriends. He became familiar with every heart surgery technique, participated in more than three hundred open-heart operations, but left America never having performed a single open-heart procedure as surgeon.

CHAPTER FOURTEEN

CAPE TOWN

I n the summer of 1958, Barnard returned to Cape Town to establish an open-heart surgery program at Groote Schuur. It would be the first such program in Africa, but the director had never, himself, performed an open-heart operation.

The beautiful southern tip of Africa was far removed from the mainstream of the world. The racial strife of apartheid and hostility between the Afrikaners and the British descendants consumed South African society, and the total absence of television added to the sense of isolation. The medical establishment traveled to Great Britain and beyond for training. As a result, the staff at Groote Schuur was well-equipped, well-trained, and generally excellent. Ancillary testing was as up-to-date, and even rudimentary cardiac catheterization was available.

Barnard, self-confident as he was, had never been captain of the ship. Now he stood at the helm without experienced hands to guide him. His seniors in cardiology, in some measure aware of this, began by presenting the simplest cases for surgery. Barnard was adept at opening the chest, running the bypass machine, and closing, which was what assistants did. He also knew chapter and verse of every procedure, so repairing atrial septal defects did not present a challenge. After the first few cases went well, more complex problems were sent his way. Soon, a variety of open-heart surgery operations were being performed weekly in Cape Town, South Africa.

Barnard was not a particularly dexterous surgeon. Some felt he was barely more than adequate and certainly not naturally gifted like Cooley. The surgeons at the University of Minnesota, brilliant and innovative as they were, had not been technical wizards either. But Barnard was hampered by rheumatoid arthritis, which often made surgery painful and challenging. The tools he brought to the table were intensity, perseverance, and superior intellect, and they would suffice in building a cardiac surgery department with exemplary results. Barnard himself would often allude to being less than a graceful surgeon, which was always meant to point out that though he was slower and less flashy, his results were superior. This he attributed to being more attentive to detail at surgery, and fastidious about post-operative patient care.

In the operating room, Barnard demanded absolute quiet, which may have been a crutch for the less gifted operator, but it also added tension to an already tense situation. The silence was not infrequently broken by Barnard's own angry outbursts directed at assistants, anesthesiologists, or pump technicians. The greater the difficulties during surgery, the more blame he ascribed to others. Boyish charm quickly turned into the lash, and highly trained assistants could not help but resent him. But Barnard demanded as much from himself as he could possibly give. If insecurity was at the root of his behavior at surgery, the same man would often sit the night at a patient's bedside. Nor was there any self-doubt evident in patient care, or at professional conferences.

Marius Barnard, five years his brother's junior, entered the world of cardiovascular surgery in the shadow of his volatile and egocentric sibling. After a year studying with the famously abusive Michael DeBakey and the smooth Denton Cooley, Marius joined the cardiac surgery group led by Christiaan, now an important heart surgeon. Christiaan always insisted on a fully trained surgeon as his assistant, and the task often fell to Marius, who considered himself far more skilled than his elder brother. The assistant role was short lived, and they quickly resumed their flinty relationship. Marius, however, consistently defended his brother's excellent results, which he too attributed to meticulous, if exceedingly slow surgery, brilliant instincts, and unmatched post-operative care. What he did not defend was having his own contributions go unacknowledged.

★ ★ ★ ★ ★

Organ transplantation became a reality on December 23rd, 1954, at the Peter Bent Brigham Hospital in Boston, when twenty-three-year-old Ronald Herrick donated a kidney to his identical twin, Richard, who was dying of chronic glomerulonephritis. The history making doctor, Joseph Murray, was a plastic surgeon who spent years treating major burns with skin grafts and was very much aware that grafts between unrelated individuals were rejected. Understanding that the Herrick twins were genetically identical, Murray assumed correctly that the transplanted organ would not be recognized as foreign, and hence, would not be rejected.

The headline-grabbing five-hour surgery was a giant step forward, but it sidestepped the rejection phenomenon that knowledgeable people, including Murray, knew was the real stumbling block. Murray, and many others, had begun experimenting with immunosuppression, using crude drugs and X-ray therapy to control rejection with varying degrees of success. The Herrick brothers provided an opportunity to demonstrate the vast possibilities in the absence of rejection.

Progress dealing with tissue rejection was excruciatingly slow until 1960, when the British immunologist Peter Medawar devised a method of tissue typing, not unlike blood typing, which helped identify closely related individuals between whom the foreign body reaction would be less violent. By 1962, the combination of tissue typing and immunosuppression was being employed for kidney transplantation, increasing survival time. For his groundbreaking work, Murray was awarded the Nobel Prize in Physiology or Medicine in 1990.

Once kidney transplantation became a reality, heart transplantation was openly discussed. Like any other organ, some hearts are diseased beyond repair. Suddenly, the glib phrase "he needs a new heart," was being taken seriously. In the early 1960s, two schools of thought were being entertained for irreparably damaged hearts: transplantation, which would build on the knowledge of kidney transplantation; and the artificial heart, which integrated technologies developed for valves, pumps, and pacemakers.

The surgical techniques of transplantation were not new. In 1950, Vladimir Demikhov accomplished ingenious feats in a Moscow cellar that resembled an unhinged surgeon run amuck. Among them was transplanting entire heads from dog to dog and creating living, two-headed dogs. It was a freaky concept, but a technical tour de force, and attracted considerable attention. Not all of it good. But he had done it and had done it repeatedly.

Demikhov was anything but unhinged; much of his work had more than shock value. As early as 1951, he transplanted dog hearts under hypothermia, cross-circulation, and even rudimentary heart-lung machines. He was also the first to note that the transplanted heart kept beating rhythmically even after its nerve supply was severed. This unexpected bit of information surfaced after he removed a dog's heart, sewed it back in place, and found the dog healthy and functional. A variation of the experiment was repeated some years later by Richard Lower, who produced a film of a dog with a transplanted heart, able to run, play, and catch a Frisbee. The additional point being the denervated heart could somehow regulate its output and perform demanding functions. Barnard was fascinated by Demikhov, and shortly after returning to South Africa in 1958, he proudly produced a two-headed dog of his own, for which he was soundly chastised when he sought publicity for the feat.

As Barnard began to ponder the possibility of heart transplantation, Marius became a critical, if uncredited player. Barnard was far from the first to take the possibility seriously, nor was he the most practiced, or the most knowledgeable. Surgeons developing techniques for heart transplantation in the dog lab were surprised to learn that the technique was not nearly as exacting as they had expected. Instruments were less specialized, suture materials and the needles used to drive the sutures were less than optimal, but the surgery could be done. For a number of technical reasons, canine cardiac surgery was more complicated than human surgery, and if it could be done in dogs, it could be done in man. That much had was clear. The issue was rejection.

The early 1960s saw long-term kidney transplant survival reaching 50 percent. David Hume, one of Murray's seniors at the Brigham, moved on to become the chief of surgery at the Medical College of Virginia. Hume and his team were responsible for great technical and theoretical advances in the discipline, including identifying basic causes for rejection in tissue and blood group typing, and new methods for the preservation of the organ from harvest to transplantation. Transplantation was transplantation, and by the mid-1960s, Hume was ready to apply what he learned from kidney transplantation to heart transplantation. What he needed was an experienced cardiac surgeon to lead the effort.

Numerous surgeons were reporting early laboratory efforts at heart transplantation. Hume was aware that the most notable progress was being made by Norman Shumway and Richard Lower at Stanford. Hume recruited Lower, offering him his own clinical division, laboratories, funding, and encouragement. The combination of Hume's expertise in managing rejection along with Lower's laboratory heart transplant experience instantly made the Medical College of Virginia a serious contender in the race to transplant the human heart. Despite universal denials from all contenders, it was, in fact, a race.

The de facto leader and spokesman for the field was Norman Shumway. An interesting, low-key iconoclast, Shumway was a delightful man with a wicked sense of humor and a single-minded quest for excellence. With and without Lower, he had performed three hundred and fifty experimental transplants with increasing success, and he was the man to beat. Lower and Shumway continued to communicate and share ideas; they were as close as competing horses in the same race could be.

In the Northeast was Adrian Kantrowitz, a big burly man who seemed most unlikely to be performing delicate cardiac surgery on tiny infants. Kantrowitz was innovative, hard-driving, and led a crack team at Maimonides Hospital, a little-known community hospital in Brooklyn.

Both Shumway and Barnard were Lillehei alumni. Lillehei himself, the founding maverick of open-heart surgery, hadn't entered the race. The year 1967 had been rough for him. His life was imploding around him and he was busy scrambling to hold it together.

Others were preparing to move ahead as well. At the University of Mississippi, James Hardy had already made head-lines and endured considerable public scorn, with the short-lived transplantation of a Chimpanzee heart into a human. Hardy underestimated the cost to his reputation and wasn't about to assume any further risk.

It was now all about rejection, and by the mid-1960s, control of the rejection phenomenon was still nowhere near accomplished. But fiddling with cocktails of powerful steroids, azathioprine, and other immunosuppressive drugs had signifi-cantly extended human kidney transplant longevity as well as heart transplants in the lab. At the forefront of progress in immunosuppression were Tom Starzl in Denver, David Hume, and Richard Lower in Richmond, and Shumway in Palo Alto.

From the outset, the likelihood of rejection was the gorilla in the room, but the most immediate hurdles were ethical. Everyone agreed that the need to replace a nonfunctioning, irreparable heart was real. The inescapable alternative was death. At some point in the decline of the moribund heart patient, the choice would be to accept the hand one had been dealt, or gamble on a new lease on life. The situation was not unlike the decision to do the first open-heart surgery a decade earlier. Even without history to help weigh the chances of success, there would still be no dearth of patients willing to roll the dice on a new heart. The problem was the donor.

Kidney transplantation was far less ethically charged simply because a living donor could function normally with the single remaining kidney. If a kidney transplant failed, the patient could resume dialysis, buy time, and go on living. Another match was possible, another attempt feasible. A kidney, cooled and flushed with blood, proved to survive well from harvest to implantation. But the human heart, all fragile, oxygen-consuming muscle, was another matter.

When the heart stops beating, blood stops flowing to the coronary arteries and the oxygen-demanding muscle mass begins to degenerate. Animal experiments confirmed the inverse relationship between time elapsed from harvest to transplant and the likelihood of success. The longer the interval, the less likely survival. Hundreds of living canine hearts had been harvested, immediately transplanted into the recipients, and lived. But both dogs had been in the operating lab. Both anesthetized, the recipient prepared and kept alive on the heart-lung machine, the donor sacrificed, and the heart immediately transplanted, eliminating the variable of time.

Exploring the issue of elapsed time, Richard Lower removed the heart of a deceased human, warmed it, perfused it with blood for a short time, and resuscitated it. Then he harvested hearts from deceased humans, warmed and perfused them, and transplanted them into baboons. The animals survived for several days before rejection.

The point had been made. A deceased heart could be warmed, perfused, and successfully transplanted. But it was more complicated than that. In actual human to human transplants, blood group and tissue typing are critical for survival. Therefore, the availability of matched donor and recipient, as well as timing, were all important factors. And these were not easy criteria to meet. A closely matched, beating heart, ready for donation, was optimal. But then there was the ethical issue.

The chain of events for kidney and heart transplantation are very similar, except—and this is a big exception—removing a beating heart from a human donor meant sacrificing the donor, which, in the most basic terms, could be considered murder. But once the potential donor's heart stopped beating, the criterion of death was met, the heart could be legally "harvested," and the letter of the law would be met.

Despite Lower's experimental evidence to the contrary, the conventional wisdom was that the period between when the heart stopped beating and when it was harvested and transplanted would cause too much damage for viability. Lower was confident that he could maintain the donor heart undamaged for a short period and transplant it successfully. But finding a matched heart nearby would require more coincidence than planning. As it happened, circumstances arose in which Lower could test his thesis when he obtained permission to harvest the heart of a terminally ill patient who had been allowed to die.

Lower was poised to be the first man to transplant a human heart, but a blood group mismatch, known from the outset, made the possibility of long-term success extremely unlikely. Despite encouragement to move forward, he declined and decided to wait for more optimal conditions.

Surgeons were technically prepared to proceed but struggled with the definition of death. Defined by the absence of
brain activity, everything would have been simpler. The donor
heart could continue beating until it stopped at the moment
of transplant. Or, if Lower was correct, a short time before
transplant. But that was not the case, and circumstances where
matched donor and recipient were in close enough proximity to wait for the moment of death was exceedingly unlikely.
Surgeons were shackled unless they were willing to defy the
law—or find some way around it.

Shumway thought he saw a way to slip the shackles. In
November of 1967, he published his intentions as the world
of cardiovascular surgery watched. His unspoken strategy was
for the neurology team to declare brain death, disconnect the
patient from the artificial life support, ventilator, and medications, finish rounds and return half an hour later. Finding the
patient pulseless, they would declare death. It was fuzzy, but not
overtly illegal.

Before Shumway announced his intentions, Barnard had
already learned the basic techniques of heart transplantation.
The number of transplants performed in the labs at Groote
Schuur was never formally reported, but Marius Barnard estimated it at between twenty and thirty, most of which he himself had performed. Christiaan Barnard did a few, but he was
more interested in the problem of rejection and managed to
get himself invited to spend the last three months of 1966 with
Hume and Lower at the Medical College of Virginia. The visit
was ostensibly to learn the latest immunosuppression techniques for his new kidney transplantation program. Marius
Barnard was in America at the same time, taking a year of post
graduate cardiovascular training in Houston, and briefly visited

Richmond while his brother was in residence. Barnard's former pump technician from Groote Schuur had moved to America and joined Lower's team in Virginia as well. In a moment of old country comradery, Barnard let his intentions slip to his former team member, saying, "I'm bloody well going to do this." But he never mentioned his plan to Lower or Hume.

As far as the Americans knew, Barnard was interested in rejection as it applied to his kidney transplant program, and Marius was just passing through. All evidence points to this not having been the case. In fact, upon returning home, Barnard performed a total of just one kidney transplant. Hardly the impression he had left with his hosts in Virginia.

His engaging, outgoing personality and sharp, quick wit, made Barnard well-liked at the Medical College of Virginia. He was not in charge of anything, did not have his operative skills tested, and he hadn't the opportunity to lose his temper or castigate underlings. His family was in Cape Town, and he had no responsibilities in Virginia. He was learning what he needed to learn and there were no restrictions on having a good time. He partied, met new women, and planned his route to fame.

Lower did not consider Barnard a threat, and Barnard did nothing to dispel that image.

Barnard returned to Cape Town in December of 1966, bringing with him the accumulated knowledge of the world's experts in immunosuppression. It was full steam ahead through 1967. Though technically less well-prepared, Barnard was in a slightly better position than his American counterparts to make the attempt. The issue of absent brain inactivity as the definition of death had not been argued in South Africa, and there was no legal opposition to doing so.

★ ★ ★ ★ ★

The Barnard family home was in a lakeside community, an easy half-hour drive from the hospital, and far enough removed to be out of the mainstream. Barnard worked late nights at the hospital, and suitably distanced from his family, continued his pattern of extra marital affairs. The time he did spend at home was obsessively devoted to his daughter, Diedre, a world-class water skier and the apple of her father's watchful eye. It was not what most would consider a normal life.

Barnard concentrated a great deal of his time on the transplant team and ramped up to full alert once Shumway announced his intentions. In addition to technicians, nurses, and a cardiologist, the small group included an immunologist, even though Barnard himself was fully conversant in the drug routines employed by Hume. Plans remained closely held and other Groote Schuur surgeons were intentionally excluded. Weekly strategy meetings continued, and the search for a heart recipient intensified. He was found in the person of Louis Washkansky.

Washkansky was a big-hearted man with very little left of his heart. A fifty-three-year-old smoking, drinking, fun-loving, diabetic, he had suffered massive heart damage due to coronary artery disease. The damage to his heart muscle led to severe congestive heart failure, and his enlarged, inefficient heart left him chronically short of breath and his limbs bloated with edema. By December of 1967, Washkansky was unable to function and near death. When Barnard introduced the possibility of attempting a transplant, Washkansky recognized both the inherent risk in this unproven operation and the fact that it was the only thing between him and imminent death.

The high-living wholesale grocer was a terrible transplant candidate, and therefore a patient who needed it most. Barnard was aware of Washkansky's tenuous grasp on life; healthy people didn't need to have their hearts replaced. Attempts had been made to reduce the edema fluid collected in Washkansky's legs by inserting drainage catheters, which became infected, an element that Barnard may have underestimated. As Washkansky weakened, and a proper donor failed to materialize, he began to abandon hope.

Then, on December 2, 1967, a pleasant, South African summer Sunday, at 3:45 p.m., Denise Darvall, and her mother, Myrtle, were crossing a busy street carrying a cake for a teatime visit to a friend's home. Almost to their parked car filled with family members, the two women were struck by a speeding car. Myrtle Darvall was killed instantly. Twenty-five-year-old Denise suffered multiple serious injuries, and later that day, was declared brain dead by three neurologists in the ICU at Groote Schuur Hospital. At this point, the family was approached, consented to organ donation, and the transplant team assembled. Barnard was at home when the call came and preparations were already being made as they had been laid out in the weekly prep meetings: donor and recipient were placed in adjoining operating rooms; surgeons and nurses in sterile green gowns, white caps, and green masks stood at their stations; and Barnard was in the room with Darvall. When she was declared brain dead, her heart still beating, he was ready to proceed. At truly the last minute, Barnard refused to use brain death alone to allow him to take Denise Darvall's heart. Despite pressure from all involved, he hesitated, as though suddenly understanding the implications. Finally, he moved to the head of the table and disconnected the ventilator. Denise Darvall ceased breathing, her heart fibrillated and stopped beating. By any and all measures, she was dead.

Satisfied, Barnard personally harvested her heart. It was quickly connected to a heart-lung machine and perfused with cooled, oxygenated blood and carried into the room where Louis Washkansky lay anesthetized, connected to another heart-lung bypass machine. Then, the difficulties began.

A perfusion cannula placed in Washkansky's femoral artery malfunctioned due to the sclerotic nature of the compromised vessel. This required the catheter from the heart-lung machine to be removed and placed in his aorta instead. That completed, Barnard looked around the room and gave the order.

"Clamp the line."

In the excitement, he hadn't preceded the order with "pump off." The machine perfusing Washkansky had been left running, and as pressure built, it fractured the arterial line. Blood wildly sprayed all over the room. In a shower of blood, Barnard realized what had happened.

"Cut the pump, cut the pump." Barnard shouted, and then berated the nurse who had simply followed his orders. Everyone in the room had been aware of where the fault lay. Barnard rallied immediately and pulled the line from Washkansky before his system was suffused with lethal air. When the mistake was corrected, the system had to be reprimed with blood to purge the tubing of air bubbles. By this point, Barnard's tremor had become almost uncontrollable. To make matters worse, not a single one of his assistants for the historic procedure in operating room 2A had ever witnessed, much less performed, a heart transplant in the animal lab. No one knew the drill. One of Barnard's primary assistants, a competent and reliable surgeon, had been unaware that the momentous procedure was contemplated.

The sternum splitting incision in Washkansky's chest was held wide open by mechanical retractors. Still shaky, Barnard removed the massively enlarged heart and struggled to replace it with the comparatively tiny heart of a healthy twenty-five-year-old woman—a walnut in a coconut shell.

To make matters worse, the donor heart, which had been cooled to preserve it, did not immediately begin beating. Moments of silent horror filled the room each time the pump was turned off and nothing happened. The room filled with the loudest imaginable silence, until finally, on the third try, Denise Darvall's heart began to beat rhythmically in Louis Washkansky's chest. His blood pressure began to rise toward normal, and happy murmurs filled the room. Christiaan Barnard reached across the table and shook the bloody, gloved hand of his assistant, just as Walt Lillehei had done at the completion of Gregory Glidden's operation.

Under these astounding circumstances, Barnard had persevered, and five hours later, he had completed the world's first successful human heart transplant. Barnard had planned for this moment. He had previously informed the Minister of the Interior of the impending operation, and he had succeeded. He had succeeded despite not having prepared in the manner of Shumway, Lower, or Kantrowitz. He succeeded despite an abysmally unsuccessful laboratory transplant record, and without a rigorously-trained surgical team. He was determined to be first. He was first, and he basked in his glory.

When informed, Shumway, the master of the technique, commented, "Barnard, of all people." He would not be the only cardiac surgeon to utter the phrase.

Cooley, on the other hand, wired Barnard.

"Congratulations on your first heart transplant, Chris. I will soon be doing my one hundredth. Denton Cooley."

★　★　★　★　★

The avalanche of media coverage was unlike anything even Barnard himself had anticipated. While there was every likelihood he had leaked his plans, he was unprepared for journalists surrounding the hospital, blocking entrances, crawling the halls, and breaching protocols trying to reach Louis Washkansky and his now famous surgeon. Barnard modestly acclaimed teamwork, but his scientific reports, contrary to long precedent, had only one author: Christiaan Barnard.

Television networks from around the world sought him and he quickly accepted an invitation to the United States for a major interview on *Face the Nation*. Much as he sought the limelight, he was shocked that there was no respite from reporters. The Barnard family resorted to sleeping away from home to escape the endless personal intrusions and phone calls in an attempt to find some desperately needed sleep. Finally, Groote Schuur assigned a team to issue regular status reports on the world's first heart transplant patient, and the South African government saw an opportunity to put on a good face for the world. Opposition to apartheid had been building globally, and this was an opportunity for good press among the community of nations. Little was known of South Africa, less of Cape Town, and nothing at all of Groote Schuur. It is not much of an exaggeration to say that Barnard had put his hospital, and his city, on the map.

Initially, Washkansky did quite well. With an endotracheal breathing tube, a urinary catheter, continuous blood transfusions, intravenous fluids, and blood pressure and venous pressure monitoring, his condition, though critical, was promising. His physicians monitored these signals, watched the massive swelling of his legs disappear as the efficient new heart did its work, and marveled at his steady, rhythmic heartbeat.

After four days of steady improvement, his endotracheal tube was removed and he could speak. A few short interviews were permitted, and Washkansky showered praise on Barnard, who had achieved the goal he had once confided to DeBakey; he was now a world-famous surgeon.

★ ★ ★ ★ ★

In Brooklyn, three days after the Washkansky operation, Adrian Kantrowitz made his attempt transplanting an infant heart. The recipient lived just six hours after surgery. Kantrowitz performed the surgery in less than an hour, under hypothermia and without bypass. There was speculation that a faulty rewarming process had resulted in metabolic changes causing the cessation of the heartbeat. Kantrowitz considered the operation a failure. He had actually been prepared to precede Barnard by six months when the first operation was aborted by hospital administrators on the sticky question of brain death versus absent heartbeat. The ultimate irony was Barnard's last-minute decision to wait for cardiac death before proceeding.

A year after the Barnard breakthrough, medical ethicists redefined death to coincide with absence of brain function. Meanwhile, surgeons devised ways to maintain the viability of the donor heart after cardiac death, all of which had worked in the favor of Barnard. He was there first, and he wasn't about to stop.

Shumway performed his first heart transplant a month after Barnard. The patient survived only fifteen days. Five months later, Cooley performed his first transplant.

★ ★ ★ ★ ★

Seven days after surgery, Washkansky began to weaken significantly. On the twelfth post-operative day, he developed a high fever. A chest X-ray revealed cloudy infiltrates that Barnard likened to a condition he had seen in Hume's kidney transplant patients. Hume had called it Transplant Lung. Barnard, taking his cue from Hume, treated it with additional azathioprine, the primary and most potent of immunosuppressants. In fact, Washkansky had developed pneumonia, not the rejection phenomenon. The massive antibiotic therapy that followed failed to correct the downhill course. Treating Louis Washkansky with additional immunosuppressants had crippled his ability to fight off the infection that had likely been seeded from his infected leg catheters, and ultimately led to his death on the eighteenth post-operative day.

Barnard had become an international hero. He was heavily invested in his patient's survival, pulled out all stops, and had done his best in a situation with no obvious precedent to follow. The pride he felt on seeing his face on the covers of both *Time* and *Life* magazines was now tainted, but there was no stopping the avalanche of publicity. The public still considered him a miracle worker, and the hero worship train carried a privately saddened but optimistic Barnard on a whirlwind trip, which he increasingly managed to enjoy.

Following Jewish tradition, Louis Washkansky's funeral was held on the day after his death. For unknown reasons, Barnard did not attend. The arrangements he made with CBS soon had him in New York, where, a few days after Washkansky's death, he visited his friend and mentor, Walt Lillehei, now professor and surgeon in chief at the New York Hospital-Cornell University Medical Center. After speaking to a packed house at surgical grand rounds, Barnard presented Lillehei with a signed copy of the *Time* cover in which Lillehei's face replaced Barnard's in the picture. Chris and Louwtjie Barnard spent a glamorous Christmas at the Plaza Hotel in New York. He was the toast of the town. So exalted was his new status that an Air Force plane was assigned to meet his travel needs. The Barnards lunched with President and Mrs. Lyndon Johnson in Texas, and then went on to visit with Cooley, where he was brought back to earth by the fun-loving Cooley who greeted him on the red carpet.

"Hi, Boy. What's your name?"

The tour was a grand success enjoyed by the overwhelmed couple who had last been in America together, living hand to mouth in Minneapolis.

★   ★   ★   ★   ★

Before Louis Washkansky's death, the cardiology team at Groote Schuur had already identified a second candidate for transplant. Philip Blaiberg, a fifty-eight-year-old dentist was barely surviving therapy resistant heart failure secondary to coronary artery disease, a situation not unlike Washkansky's. Blaiberg remained optimistic and committed to the surgery even after learning of

Washkansky's death. It was his only hope for survival, and he clung to it.

While Barnard was off charming the world, giving interviews, appearing on panel shows, and fielding questions about the ethics of transplantation, the cardiology team at Groote Schuur had been on the lookout for a suitable donor for Blaiberg. What they would have done if a donor had been identified while Barnard was still on his publicity tour is unknown. Marius was at least as qualified as his brother to perform the surgery, but would it have been permitted? In any event, shortly after Barnard's return, Clive Haupt, a twenty-four-year-old man of mixed race, was declared brain dead of a massive cerebral hemorrhage.

The weary Barnard was on hand and in the operating room on January 2, 1968. Although his team now had transplant experience under their belts, the second surgery was not a picture-perfect exercise either. Despite a few stumbles, Blaiberg did well. Some important lessons had been learned from their first experience. A sterile, isolation room was provided, and a physician from Barnard's staff was there full-time to monitor, manage, and prevent infection and rejection. Recovery was slow, but positive, and on the seventy-first post-operative day, Philip Blaiberg became the first heart transplant recipient ever to leave the hospital. Media attention once again verged on hysteria. There were television and book contracts for the patient, leaked photographs and stories, but in general, things had been far better organized.

Barnard, despite having denied intentionally igniting the firestorm of attention surrounding his first surgery, was afforded every opportunity by a fawning media to build his own legend. Blaiberg helped. His every move toward a normal life was chronicled, and he missed no opportunity to laud the surgeon who had given him new life, and even wrote a book about it. Accounts of his "normal" life included repeated stories of Barnard presenting him with his actual heart, which he had held and written about. Photographs of Blaiberg frolicking in the Cape Town surf were front-page news. Some observers, independent of publicity releases, painted a picture of a frail man being helped in and out of the sea. However vital or frail Blaiberg had been, this was a man living with another man's heart beating in his chest and did much to portray heart transplantation in a hopeful and positive light. In truth, this was to be the exception, not the rule.

Transplants performed during this period by Shumway, Lower, and Kantrowitz had not fared nearly so well. Most died in the immediate post-operative period, or shortly thereafter, usually from acute rejection. What had been proven was that the operation was possible, and was, in fact, more of an ethical, logistic, and immunological problem than a surgical challenge. With the fear and newness factor behind them, there was little talk of technical difficulties among the surgeons. Cooley was doing his transplants with fewer than forty minutes on the pump and less than an hour from "skin to skin," as surgeons measure time spent from beginning to end of an operation. There were, and would be, two very basic problems limiting the value and ubiquity of heart transplants: First and foremost, the rejection phenomenon. Second, and unsolved to this day, the inadequate supply of donors to serve the multitude of failing hearts.

For two years after the Washkansky operation, heart transplants were no longer medical news. Cooley, the most prolific operator, performed twenty transplants in a sixteen month period, with only two long-term survivors. Soon, transplant deaths would result in a virtual moratorium on the procedure for a decade. But in 1968, the euphoria was gaining momentum.

Six months after his surgery, Blaiberg began to show signs of rejection. The episode was controlled by the team's first use of anti-lymphocyte serum, a new immunosuppressive tool. Blaiberg rallied and did well until he began to develop significant coronary artery disease in his twenty-five-year-old heart, an unexpected condition soon to be recognized as a sign of chronic rejection. The progressive nature of the occlusion of the coronary arteries was potentially lethal, and its rapid progress in the face of no known therapy raised the prospect of a second transplant, which was rejected.

Philip Baliberg died nineteen months after receiving his new heart. His name and his odyssey were known around the globe. By the time of Blaiberg's death, Christiaan Barnard had moved fully onto the world stage, changed his life, wrecked his marriage, gratified his ego, and achieved the fame he had so single-mindedly sought.

Correspondence, telephone calls, and invitations for professional and social appearances overwhelmed the ability of the hospital to cope. Groote Schuur had neither a public relations department, nor consultants, and a single secretary was assigned to deal with the mountains of mail and requests for Barnard's presence, which were sorted and organized for the professor's consideration.

Barnard's travel was no longer at his own expense or hampered by the limited budget of the hospital. The South African government now paid for first-class air travel and provided a car and driver for his official use. Barnard estimated he had flown a quarter of a million miles in the year following his first transplant. If nothing else, he was the good face of South Africa. His personal antipathy to apartheid was personal. He did not advertise his opposition on his travels, nor did he make any effort to condone it. Despite the occasional assault on the policies of his homeland, Barnard was the finest, most sought-after, articulate, intelligent, and charming ambassador the increasingly ostracized country could have dreamed of. For much of the world, Christiaan Barnard had become South Africa, and South Africa had brought the world the miracle of heart transplantation. Barnard had begun to believe it as well.

★　★　★　★　★

On his first post-transplant victory tour, Barnard was his usual disheveled, boyish, forty-five-year-old self. Travelling in rumpled old suits, unstarched shirts, and often without underwear, he arrived as the charming country boy made good, and the world welcomed him as a celebrity. On his second European trip, some weeks after the Blaiberg surgery, the country boy had already fallen in love with the elegance of bespoke Italian tailoring and stylish Gucci shoes. By the time he had taken his Papal audience, he presented the image of a man of the world. But whether in threadbare trousers or fine, ten-ounce, worsted wool suits, Barnard remained the witty, smiling, and irrepressible character who won new friends as easily as his ill-tempered, self-serving behavior had lost them among his coworkers.

Unusually open and freewheeling in public, the now famous surgeon, grown up in a world without television, was totally unpretentious and at ease in front of the camera. His oddly handsome features were photogenic. His boyish, toothy grin was ready and disarming. His longish, dark hair receding a bit, was combed over from left to right, and he wore a modest version of the sideburns popular at the moment. Interviewers were charmed. Even the "hard" questions were softballs, and he was obviously delighted to be at the center of it all.

On this second victory lap, Barnard traveled alone. Well-dressed and perpetually tanned, he was entirely at ease with a cigarette in one hand and a drink in the other. A photograph with an enraptured Sophia Loren, with whom he was alleged to have slept, was widely circulated. He danced publicly to the beginning of a much-publicized affair with Gina Lollobrigida and proceeded to take Europe by storm. The popular press covered Barnard having a grand time. All of this was followed closely and unhappily at home. Louwtjie, who had managed to ignore, or perhaps forgive, her husband's serial infidelities, was embarrassed for herself and their teenaged son and daughter.

After all the publicity from Europe, Louwtjie accompanied Barnard on a trip to San Francisco. Just before he was scheduled to lecture, Barnard asked her to run back to their hotel room to fetch slides he had forgotten. Rummaging through his brief case, she found a love letter from Lollobrigida. For Louwtjie, it was the final insult.

Shortly thereafter, Barnard returned from a solo European trip and found all his worldly possessions packed into the official car that met him at the airport. The marriage was over. It was the end of the first of three failed marriages, and multiple, well-publicized affairs with beautiful, young women.

★ ★ ★ ★ ★

On each of his whirlwind world tours, Barnard took part in discussions with the other transplant pioneers, each of whom he treated with winning respect. Only Shumway made it his business to avoid the man whom he felt had not earned his stripes in the lab, learned other's secrets by subterfuge, and succeeded under false pretenses. Lower, the other pioneer who had reason to feel used, spoke negatively of Barnard's personal aggrandizement and self-serving devotion to the use of the pronoun *I*, where *we* would have been more appropriate. Cooley, no shrinking violet in the ego department, liked and respected Barnard. DeBakey, neither a contemporary, nor a competitor, liked and respected him as well, and Lillehei, who trained him, liked Barnard very much. And there was a great deal to like—if one wasn't too close.

By no measure was Barnard a great surgeon. He was slow, tense, unsure, suffered a tremor, painful, and had increasingly deformed, rheumatoid hands. Even though his few experimental transplants had done poorly, his human heart transplants had by far the best long-term outcomes of all the practitioners. Of his first six transplant patients, one had survived for thirteen years, and another for more than two decades, a record unmatched when the only immunosuppressives were azathioprine, steroids, and anti-lymphocyte serum. All who worked for and with Barnard attributed this to innately superb clinical judgement and obsessive work habits, assets that even his harshest critic, his increasingly estranged brother, Marius, would not deny. He was special. He was a risk-taker. He was difficult. He was an insensitive taskmaster, and a brilliant opportunist devoted to his patients. But life was getting in the way of his work.

CHAPTER FIFTEEN

FAMOUS

S hortly after the great Blaiberg success, Barnard assumed the life of the international celebrity he had become. He lectured more and operated less. His staff at Groote Schuur kept the department functioning, and the professor, tired and distracted, operated in spurts between engagements, soon performing only two or three procedures per week, and the occasional transplant. Still, the cardiovascular service at the hospital was operating at capacity. Barnard had become the legendary rainmaker, and patients from Africa and beyond sought his care, most of which was handed down to his staff.

By 1970, enthusiasm for heart transplants waned as it became clear that surgeons were losing the battle to organ rejection. Barnard's transplant practice dwindled to nearly none, Cooley quit, and Kantrowitz had long since moved on to artificial heart assistance devices and artificial hearts. DeBakey performed a dozen surgeries and quit, more convinced than ever that the future was the artificial heart. Lillehei did several transplants and a dramatic simultaneous heart and lung transplant. Shumway persevered, juggled antirejection medi-cations, and gradually achieved increasing longevity for his patients. Most centers saw the writing on the wall and declared a moratorium on the costly, unpredictable procedure, with its all-too-rare successes. The bloom was off the rose and would remain dormant for a decade until a new immunosuppressive drug was discovered.

In May of 1969, Barnard was divorced by Louwtjie. On Valentine's Day of 1970, he married Barbara Zoellner, a beau-tiful, nineteen-year-old heiress, and a contemporary of his daughter, Diedre.

On their extended honeymoon trip, the couple planned to visit the Cooley's in Houston. Cooley advised Barnard that he would be most welcome, and he would invite his daughter's friends so the bride would feel at home.

Despite the twenty-nine-year age gap, the marriage pros-pered. Financially, Barnard continued on his modest govern-ment salary, half of which was devoted to alimony and child support. But the financial situation was eased by a generous allowance Barbara received from her father, who also bought an upscale home for them. The clamor to hang on Barnard's every word made his memoir, *One Life*, written with a ghost writer, an international bestseller. Barnard designated the income from the book to a foundation supporting heart disease research and surgery. He would later joke that had he known how much money the book would generate, he would not have given the rights away.

Barbara, a confident, socially connected young woman, was perfectly comfortable in her husband's high-flying world. The couple had two children, and a very public life. Barnard, however, continued his affairs, and, in 1980, after ten years of marriage, they, too, divorced.

The early eighties gave the first hints of a headlong slide from the top of the world. Suffering the loss of a woman he apparently loved deeply, Barnard acknowledged his misbehavior publicly. In a second memoir, he claimed that Barbara had had an affair with a younger man, while he, the great Christiaan Barnard, endured the painful, deformed hands and immobility of rheumatoid arthritis.

As early as a decade after his historic surgery, Barnard had begun looking for reasons to avoid surgery. The hospital was drudgery, surgery was torment, his arthritis had worsened, and he wanted a different life. In December of 1983, wearing the public face of a martyr, he retired from the University of Cape Town and cardiac surgery. By his own admission, the reasons for withdrawal were less physical than a loss of interest in operating.

Barnard qualified for a full salary government pension, but it was not nearly enough to support the lifestyle to which he had become accustomed. With no interest in returning to the simple life, and an adoring public, there were endless opportunities for the famous Christiaan Barnard.

Tragedy struck in 1984 with the death of Andre, Barnard's son with Louwtjie. A pediatrician with a known drug problem, the young man was found overdosed and drowned in his bathtub. The loss struck hard, and there was public soul searching on Barnard's part as he dealt with it. His daughter, Diedre, had consumed his family time, at the expense of Andre, and his recriminations surfaced altogether too late. It was a particularly difficult time as every event in Barnard's life was still being chronicled publicly. Private mourning was not an option.

In the transition from surgeon to public figure, Barnard became an all-purpose guru. He began a long-running, wide-ranging, syndicated newspaper column, authored another memoir—a book on dealing with rheumatoid arthritis—and authored numerous novels, all with either significant editorial help, or ghost writers. And if his books weren't particularly noteworthy, the market for them was.

After retiring from surgery Barnard accepted a position at the Baptist Medical Center in Oklahoma City, Oklahoma. It was a time of renewed interest in transplants, and the advisory post was designed to help build a new program and garner publicity for the effort. Barnard, and the head of the program, Nazih Zuhdi, had crossed paths when they were both training with Lillehei. The effort was successful for Zudhi, and remunerative for Barnard. For two years of part-time work, he was paid more than twenty times his annual government salary.

Not all the opportunities presented to Barnard were as simple and transparent, and he found his next life as the spokesperson for the dubious Clinique La Prairie in Switzerland. The clinic catered to wealthy patrons seeking to regain youth and vitality from the injection of fetal sheep cells. Barnard was careful to dance around the question of efficacy. The scientific community was more than skeptical, and after years of injecting the rich and famous, the procedure was banned. But if there was no evidence of efficacy, there was enough basic science for Barnard to defend. And he was very well paid.

Then Barnard made another disastrous leap into bed with the same entrepreneurs. This time, they were promoting a rejuvenating skin cream called Glycel. Again, Barnard stuck to the science, speaking only of what the magic ingredient could do in the lab. But try as he might to avoid it, and he seems not to have tried terribly hard, Glycel became Dr. Barnard's cream. It was expensive and sales were great. But as Barnard filled his pockets, he suffered irreparable damage to his reputation. Fronting for clinics, useless creams, and paid public speaking filled Barnard's days, but he was finally financially well off. His second memoir sold well, as did many of his total of eleven novels and books of advice. He was famous, but tarnished.

The international media darling, Christiaan Barnard, slipped further from the pedestal after a scathing interview with the British television host, David Frost, who all but blamed him as personally responsible for the apartheid. Barnard tried to arrange a return bout for which he was prepared, but Frost declined. Barnard retreated to South Africa, where he was known for his lifelong anti-apartheid stance. He purchased a 30,000 acres game farm and met the blonde, beautiful, and very young Karin Setzkorn. They married in 1988, when he was sixty-five, and she was twenty-one. The couple had two children, and Barnard, out of the limelight, and generally unscheduled, spent a great deal of time with his young family. Despite a rewarding home life, he was still unsettled. He traveled whenever invited, gained weight, suffered facial skin cancers, maintained his youthful appearance with the help of cosmetic surgery, and continued his habitual womanizing. He and Karen were divorced in September of 2000.

In September of 2001, seventy-eight-year-old Christiaan Neethling Barnard, the most famous doctor in the world, died of an acute asthma attack while vacationing on Cyprus.

CHAPTER SIXTEEN

MINNEAPOLIS

B y 1962, Walt Lillehei passed the milestone of his thousandth open-heart surgery. Not yet fifty, he had trained many of the leading surgeons in the field and befriended or mentored others. In 1955, his standing in the profession rose when, along with Varco, Warden, and Cohen, he won the Albert Lasker Award for his contribution to medical science. The prestigious award was considered the American Nobel Prize. By the early 1960s, the nay-saying older generation could no longer ignore him, and Lillehei's wild ideas became the basic tenets of the discipline. He was the President of the American College of Cardiology and a sought-after speaker.

Valve replacement surgery was born in this period, and Lillehei's contributions were a mixed bag of spectacular successes and abject failure. His work replacing diseased mitral valves had been a dramatic success. His technique differed from that of others in that he insisted on leaving a section of the old valve in place to provide infrastructure. His surgical results were the best in the country, a mortality rate of only 9.3 percent.

Kirklin, at Mayo, reported 14–20 percent mortality, and the rest of the world the same, or worse. Lillehei was instinctively certain of a technique that survives as the standard today.

Aortic valve replacement surgery was another story. With an abysmal 39 percent mortality rate, it was flat out the worst in the world. Stubborn, Lillehei altered his techniques a bit, seemingly oblivious to the loss of life.

With the development of coronary bypass surgery later in the decade, Lillehei was not the surgical superstar he had been, largely due to his failing eyesight. He had begun to develop premature cataracts, accelerated by his radiation therapy and exposure in his lab work. His surgical performance suffered, and his obstinacy and immunity to criticism had begun to work against him.

On the positive side, the DeWall-Lillehei bubble oxygenator was a commercial success, as was the next generation, a membrane type oxygenator. The portable defibrillator, artificial heart valves, and other innovations were in every cardiac operating room and intensive care unit in the world. Despite donating all royalties to the university, a sum estimated to be many tens of millions of dollars, Lillehei was well off financially. His stake in Medtronic had grown exponentially, his practice flourished, and his investments grew beyond his imagination. He and Kaye maintained a busy social life and a lively family life with four children. The Lillehei's were members of the country club, they bought a riverside home in St. Paul and a fancy speedboat, each drove a Cadillac, and Lillehei continued to indulge his taste for flashy clothing and gold jewelry.

Lillehei had a unique presence and an air of intensity about him. The cancer surgery had stripped the muscles from his neck and the scalding radiation left him with a fixed cant of his head to the right that gave the appearance of constant discomfort. But there was never a hint of awareness or self-pity in his demeanor. As a sought-after speaker for medical meetings, his general rule remained that he would take on no more than four meetings a year. But when he did attend a meeting, he was often the last man at the bar, and often did not leave alone. Cooley, with whom he developed a firm friendship, offered the advice, "never try to drink with Lillehei."

The department of surgery remained unchanged through the early 1960s. With Wangensteen in command, Lillehei and Varco ran cardiac surgery, and their laboratories produced a decade of enormous progress. As Wangensteen neared his seventieth birthday, he announced his intention to retire as chair of the department of surgery. Partial paralysis from an undiagnosed illness had already forced him to stop operating. Many were pleased to see the Wangensteen brand of surgery disappear, but his authority remained unchallenged. The professor had built a department steeped in the ethic of surgical research. As though he had willed it, the University of Minnesota had become the birthplace of cardiovascular surgery, and it was time for C. Walton Lillehei to assume the place held for him by his chief, who expected the transition to be natural and welcome. Wangensteen had put the department of surgery on the map, and his chosen heir had brought it unimagined glory.

Lillehei made no effort to insert himself in the contest for the chair. Running the department had never been his objective. In fact, prior to Wangensteen's retirement, Lillehei had favored Varco as chief. His reality was simply doing the work that interested him and Varco, his close friend and coworker, would understand him and not stand in his way. But Varco had apparently made enemies within the administration, and he had been eliminated as a candidate before the search for a successor had even begun.

Not wanting to see an outsider assume the chair, Lillehei changed his mind and arranged a meeting with Robert Howard, dean of the medical school, and offered himself as a candidate. Howard responded that Lillehei was not known to be interested in teaching medical students or administration and would not be the right man for the job.

Having thought the job was his for the asking, Lillehei was surprised. He responded by letter, modestly outlining his role in the development of open-heart surgery, and his administrative experience commanding a one thousand bed MASH unit in Italy.

Howard was decidedly unimpressed. He had, in fact, been quoted by two separate sources as having said, "Lillehei is an egomaniac, a woman chaser, and a drunk, and he will become chairman over my dead body."

A search committee was formed to examine one hundred qualified surgeons and present the three best candidates for consideration. The committee wanted the department to go in a new direction, rather than continuity of the Wangensteen reign. Chief among those of that opinion was Maurice Visscher, the long-standing head of the physiology department, and the same Visscher who had worked so closely with both Wangensteen and Lillehei over the years. Visscher alleged that Lillehei was "too quick to test on patients new drugs and new ideas that had not been adequately tested in the laboratory." Visscher also claimed that Lillehei was "too unpredictable and uncontrollable." Visscher was a powerful man in academic and political circles, and his opinions carried significant weight. Neither Wangensteen nor Lillehei thought the duplicitous

Visscher harbored ill will toward them after decades as colleagues. But given the opportunity to oust the only two more
significant individuals on the faculty, Visscher did not hesitate
to air what must have been long-held grievances.

The search committee formed by Howard had been a
sham, and his choice had already been predetermined. There
was no way the man synonymous with the birth of cardiac surgery at the University of Minnesota would be the new chief. In
the spring of 1967, John Najarian, a thirty-five-year-old kidney
transplant surgeon and immunologist from San Francisco, was
installed as professor and chairman.

CHAPTER SEVENTEEN

NEW YORK

Having rejected offers of professorships and chairs over the years, Lillehei was now ready to move on. Wangensteen, outraged by the proceedings, arranged a match between Lillehei and the New York Hospital-Cornell University Medical Center in New York City.

For twenty years, the distinguished surgeon, Frank Glenn, had served as chief of surgery at the hospital and chairman of the department at the medical school. He had followed the long reign of George Heuer, a disciple of Halsted, the revered father of modern American surgery. Attracting Lillehei was seen as a coup and a new direction for the conservative medical center.

Founded in 1771, the New York Hospital was overseen by a board of trustees culled from the highest perches of New York society. Wall Street bankers sat alongside the decedents of families with legendary wealth and famous names. The surgeons at the New York Hospital were primarily private practitioners who served the society in which they lived. As a group, they were exceptionally talented, often socially connected to their patient population, and generally expressed little interest in research.

Lillehei could bring a breath of fresh air into the stodgy halls and provide an entrée into cardiac surgery at the highest level. It remained to be seen how well a risk-taking heart surgeon would fit into the established order.

In Minnesota, Najarian named Varco chief of cardiac surgery. Lillehei informed his old friend Varco of his plans and invited a number of residents and junior staff members to join him in New York, where he planned to relocate his laboratory. Najarian forbade the removal of anything, claiming the laboratory equipment was University property. The wrangling continued, with Lillehei insisting his grant money funded the labs and should rightfully accompany him and his work. When Najarian drew his line in the sand, Lillehei said nothing. Instead, he and several members of his team rented three trucks, and in the dark of night, spirited off the entire contents of the laboratory. When the lab had been stripped bare, Lillehei left a single red rose in a glass beaker on the floor of the empty room. Leaving Minnesota behind, he jumped into his Jaguar XKE, and drove to New York and his new life.

Home life had become a bit more complicated for Kaye Lillehei. All the finery and spoils of success were obvious. She lived well, had her hobbies and her friends, and four bright, pleasant children. She loved her husband and understood his eccentricities. It was unlikely that she had been unaware of Lillehei's brief affairs, but somehow had managed to package them in the same box as his genius and his social indifference. Kaye, as many close to him, always sensed something naïve and pure about his unconventional behavior. Lillehei's rejection by the university had been a difficult episode and she had been happy for him when he received the offer from New York-Cornell.

But with children in school, Kaye was unwilling to give up her comfortable life in the twin cities and elected to stay behind. Lillehei left for New York with seventeen staff members, his precious laboratory equipment, and a powerful scientific reputation. He was named Lewis Atterbury Stimson professor of surgery, surgeon in chief of the New York Hospital, and chairman of the department of surgery at the Cornell University Medical College. It promised to be a lot of responsibility for a freewheeling surgeon who had absolutely no interest in the politics of university life.

★　★　★　★　★

The New York Hospital was a conservative institution that looked the part. The massive 1932 building runs two full city blocks along the East River. The Rockefeller University neighbors it to the south, the Hospital for Special Surgery to the north, and the Memorial Sloane-Kettering Cancer Center across the street. A meticulously planted curved entryway, valet parking and uniformed doormen added to the aura of the place and a long granite entry hall with a doctor's cloak room on the left and a private chapel on the right, gave way to a soaring lobby.

The operating rooms were on the tenth and eleventh floors. The larger rooms with viewing balconies were on one side and had natural light from the windows on the other. Lillehei had an operating theater in Minneapolis built with a viewing dome to accommodate the multitudes who made the pilgrimage to watch and learn from the father of open-heart surgery. He had always made it his business to make the observers feel welcome.

The New York Hospital surgical staff had high hopes and were anxious to watch Lillehei work. A steady stream of senior surgeons and residents filled his operating room and balcony. What they witnessed was an increasingly tentative surgeon happily taking on any challenge. His formerly chatter free operating rule had been replaced with music, another first at his new home. The general consensus had been that Lillehei was an adventurous risk-taker, but not a particularly good surgeon. He himself had no idea how he was perceived. That much hadn't changed.

Lillehei and his staff surgeons were among the very few salaried members of the department. The bulk of the attending surgeons had hospital offices or private offices located nearby in the wealthy Upper East Side neighborhood that the hospital served. They worked in the hospital, but not for the hospital; they worked for themselves, as private practitioners. They were operating surgeons, well-trained and talented. As a group, they performed roughly ten times the number of operations performed by the staff at the University of Minnesota. It was an entirely different environment, and it had not taken long for each to realize they had not gotten what they had expected.

Lillehei was surprised to find that there was no activity in the surgical laboratories. Surgical research was the lifeblood of the department at Minnesota. That was the first change he would institute. Surgical progress couldn't be made without surgical research.

For their part, the New York Hospital surgeons found the Minnesota group disappointingly slow surgeons, often requiring four or five times their own operating time for routine procedures. Slow surgery and excessive anesthesia time were not in the patient's best interest, and the whispering began. In the first several months of the Lillehei reign, operative mortality rose to unheard of levels. Lillehei, who must have been aware of the rising tide, chose not to discuss it. Not so the horrified senior staff and the administration.

The residents who had followed Lillehei from Minnesota were impressed by the quality of general surgery being performed by the New York Hospital surgeons, a closely knit, inbred, and quietly confident group: all male, white, Anglo-Saxon Protestants with a few Catholics and a single Jew in the mix. The sort of WASP enclave that could still exist in the multi-ethnic New York City of 1968. Most of the staff were indigenous New York Hospital residents, educated in eastern establishment schools, or the privileged south. Lillehei brought with him a mélange of seventeen surgeon scientists, including Jews, Blacks, Middle Easterners, Japanese, and Hindus. The newcomers were as easily identified in the stark white doctor's dining room on the fourteenth floor of the hospital tower as they were in the operating rooms.

Just days after arriving, the new chief got off to a dramatic start by successfully improving, though not fully curing, a desperately ill infant who had been deemed beyond surgical intervention by the current staff. By taking on the case, Lillehei had immediately drawn the battle lines. The old order was passing. Next, he set about instituting a surgical research program with the first truly active experimental labs the department of surgery had ever seen. Lillehei called the Cornell method of teaching "extremely archaic," with a "total lack of appreciation for the benefits of experimental work." He had an endless stream of ideas and projects to pursue and immediately set his staff to work. His firm belief in autonomy for the chief surgical residents was a position shared by the hospital. But it soon became evident that his lab-oriented men did not stack up. Minnesota

residents had been considered fully trained after having performed fewer than one hundred major operations. Residents
at the New York Hospital performed nearly one thousand such
surgeries. The basic problem had been the definition of one's
goals. Lillehei believed research meant progress and cared little
for the niceties of elegant surgery. That would come later. The
Cornell group believed surgeons best served the community
by performing the best possible surgery. To that point, they did
ten times the surgery in a quarter of the time, with a tenth the
mortality. It was hard for them to accept Lillehei's point of view.

In university hospitals, teaching responsibilities are primarily the province of the full-time faculty. It was expected
that they would lead conferences, conduct teaching rounds
and grand rounds, in which all department members, as well
as members of other disciplines, would discuss significant cases
and entertain guest speakers. Prior to Lillehei's arrival, Glenn
had been in absolute control of teaching and effectively an
important part of the hospital hierarchy.

Lillehei remained as disinterested in administration as ever.
He regularly missed conferences and made little effort to
befriend the powers at the medical center. He thought differently, dressed differently, and was governed by a wholly different rule book. Chairing his very first conference, he made light
of an opinion expressed by the chief of cardiology, Thomas
Killip, saying to an auditorium of starched white coats, "Come
on Tommy, you don't really believe it." Obviously meant good
naturedly, it was a sharp slap in the face of his new colleague.
But it was Lillehei being Lillehei. He thought nothing negative
about the comment, nor about Killip, and moved right along,
insensitive to the embarrassment he had caused and the fact
that one didn't behave that way at the New York Hospital.

But soon after arriving, Lillehei began making headlines, and the press was generally good. Suddenly, the New York Hospital-Cornell Medical Center was being talked about beyond the Upper East Side. Six months into his tenure, and approximately six months after his student, Christiaan Barnard, made history performing the first heart transplant, Lillehei performed his first heart transplant. The patient did not survive long, but subsequent transplants had very positive outcomes. As Lillehei built steam, he attempted feats that drew more media attention, particularly the following February when his team transplanted heart, kidneys, liver, and corneas into six recipients. This tour de force was followed by a heart and lung transplant, which received wide attention as well, but ended badly with rapid acute rejection.

Oblivious to the rumblings about his surgery and his Minnesota staff, Lillehei continued operating, working in his lab on new versions of his heart valve and the newest rage: the artificial heart. He made rounds at odd hours, often late at night, worked hard and played hard. Kaye was in St. Paul, and he was a "single" man in New York, a legendary leader in a major medical center where adoring, young people abounded.

After work, Lillehei could often be found just a few doors up East 70th street from the hospital, in a tavern, not surprisingly called The Recovery Room. His companions were often the surgical residents who were surprised and delighted to socialize with the chief. Some of his Minnesota transplants joined the party as well as nurses and assorted young women who worked at the hospital. Senior staff members did not participate. Many of the professors took trainees under their wings in a form of mentorship, but it was not the New York Hospital culture for professors to hold court at the local pubs.

* * * * *

Kaye enjoyed the life Lillehei provided, and as a family, they were there for one another. Not particularly happy with his drinking, she often joined, and rarely scolded. The year 1967 had been a tough one. There had been a fire that nearly burned down the house, Lillehei had been passed over for the chair and regularly indulged in more than his usual martinis. On a summer night of heavy drinking, he ran their new speedboat onto a sandbar on the St. Croix River, hurling Kaye into the dashboard. Kaye, a beautiful woman, required facial reconstructive surgery. Lillehei saw her through the recovery, and if he made the connection between his alcohol consumption and the accident, he had chosen to ignore it. He remained a hard-drinking family man with a double life.

By the time he left for New York, Kaye had decided to let him go his own way, uncertain whether the marriage would survive. Alone, Lillehei's bachelor behavior was ungoverned. Kaye's sporadic visits east often ended badly, once escalating to the point where Lillehei awakened the neighbors, shouting and banging on his locked door at 3:00 a.m.

Lillehei loved being around young women and had a few not very secret flings. More generally talked about was a long running affair with the woman who ran his operating room. None of this was missed by the administration.

* * * * *

The world of cardiovascular surgery had changed dramatically in the decade and a half since Lewis and Lillehei started it all. Surgery had transitioned from dealing solely with congenital heart defects, to transplants, to the biggest playing field of all: treating patients with coronary artery disease.

Bypassing three-to-four-millimeter coronary arteries is an exercise in sewing under magnification. Lillehei established an active program at the New York Hospital but watching him attempt to suture the tiny vessels was anything but impressive. His difficulty placing the fine sutures became so obvious to the senior residents that they attempted to help without offending. Lillehei knew something was wrong. He was fifty years old and losing his vision. Although he had never pinpointed the onset of his difficulties, it may, in part, have accounted for his horrendous series of aortic valve tragedies over his last few years at Minnesota. Possibly, late nights and alcohol added a degree of difficulty, but whatever the case, Lillehei at Cornell was not the surgeon he had been, and the case against him began to gather momentum.

Though his personal surgical statistics were acceptable, he was no longer a model worth emulating. The staff he brought with him from Minnesota had proven inept and dangerous by New York Hospital standards and were increasingly shunned. He spent little time teaching medical students and junior residents and a great deal of time in the lab. He skipped conferences and spoke his unfiltered opinions when he did attend. And the man who had previously limited his medical meetings to four times per year now managed to be away at conferences twenty times in the first two years of his tenure. This was unacceptable to the Cornell establishment, and unthinkable to the Lillehei of a decade ago.

Nothing made sense. A Lillehei cardiac fellow ordered two open-heart patients anesthetized simultaneously under orders from the chief, who was "in the elevator." Unusual to begin with, a scandal and a lawsuit resulted when it turned out Lillehei wasn't even in the country. One of the patients was the child of a justifiably outraged Cornell physician who led the legal action.

Totally oblivious to the rules of the game, Lillehei was stacking the deck against himself. When a committee was formed to investigate the disarray and poor surgical outcomes in the department, Lillehei testified as though he had been there to help. Blindness was clearly attributable to his character, not his cataracts.

In March of 1970, a bit more than two years after assuming the chairmanship at Cornell, Lillehei received a telephone call from Hugh Luckey, president of the medical center, informing him that he was being relieved of his position. An official letter followed. As of June 30, 1970, Lillehei was to be terminated as chairman of the department of surgery at Cornell University Medical College, and as surgeon in chief at the New York Hospital. He would be appointed surgeon in charge of the division of cardiovascular surgery and retain his position as Lewis Atterbury Stimson professor of surgery, along with his salary and benefits.

Lillehei was fifty-two years old when he was relieved of his chairmanship. He never quite understood how he had so displeased the powers at Cornell, and he steadfastly clung to the Wangensteen model of scientific surgery. His vision continued to deteriorate, his schizophrenic lifestyle remained unchanged, and though he had been unaware of it, his days as professor and surgeon in charge of cardiovascular surgery were numbered as well. Had that been all, he might have gently ridden off into the sunset, but far worse was yet to come.

CHAPTER EIGHTEEN

HOUSTON, DECEMBER 3, 1967

Denton Cooley was shocked when he heard the news. Christiaan Barnard, of all people. He ran a nice, small program in Cape Town, was a fun guy, but no one considered him a contender. Like everyone else, Cooley had expected Shumway to be first to transplant a human heart.

It was the next day that he sent off his telegram to Barnard. It was part congratulatory, part jest, and part prediction.

Cooley followed Barnard's first transplant by five months to the day. The surgery required only thirty-five minutes of pump time. The whole procedure, including ten anxious minutes shocking the heart into a normal rhythm, had taken less than an hour and a half, a far cry from the five hours the Barnard team had taken. As a precaution against infection, a nearby operating room was converted into a sterile ICU, and the patient, Everett Thomas, was wheeled there for recovery. The surgery had gone very well, but Cooley knew that the easy part was over, and the hurdles for survival lay ahead. Shumway had performed a transplant a month after Barnard, and although that surgery had also gone smoothly, the patient died fifteen days later. Cooley was cautiously optimistic, and not having the interest or experience in the immunological issues to follow, he established a team to take over.

By early morning, the St. Luke's administration announced the news. Another heart transplant had been performed in the United States, and the surgeon, Denton A. Cooley, held a news conference. As expected, the local and national press stirred another frenzy among the public. Cooley loved it. DeBakey learned the news upon his arrival at work that morning, promptly cancelled his surgical schedule for the day, and remained secreted off in his office.

Still smarting from being excluded from DeBakey's proposed transplant team, Cooley felt no need to advise DeBakey of his intentions. Days after the first transplant, Cooley did two more. Both patients died within eight days.

However, Everett Thomas, Cooley's first transplant patient, did well enough to leave the hospital. A position was secured for him in the trust department of a local bank so that he could resume life and be close enough for regular monitoring. The yardstick for measuring success was elastic, but Thomas's survival was measured in months, not days, and it was fair to call his operation the first successful heart transplant in the country. Certainly, that was Cooley's position.

Eight months after surgery, the signs of rejection became medically unmanageable. Thomas's heart was failing. Cooley considered a second heart transplant his only chance for survival. It was the first time a patient would undergo a second heart transplant. A matching donor was found, and the operation went smoothly enough, but Thomas died of overwhelming sepsis two days after surgery.

At Methodist, the DeBakey team was slow to get started, and by the time it had attempted its first transplant, Cooley had already performed nine.

★　★　★　★　★

By the end of 1968, it had become apparent that the operation was not the problem. Rejection, or infection, had killed seventy-one of the first one hundred heart transplants patients. By September of 1969, of Cooley's twenty transplants, nineteen patients—Everett Thomas having had two of the surgeries—only two of the nineteen were still living. Drama and publicity notwithstanding, the miracle of heart transplantation no longer seemed to be the answer to the problem of the irreparable heart. By 1971, the numbers had gotten worse. Only twenty-four of one hundred and sixty-seven patients had survived worldwide. In short order, most centers virtually abandoned the procedure.

The cover story of the September 17, 1971 issue of *Life* magazine was, "The Tragic Record of Heart Transplants."

Only Shumway and Lower persisted. Painstakingly, both groups refined immunosuppression techniques and post-operative care, and their survival rates slowly improved. But it would be another decade before rejection was tamed enough to make long-term survival a reasonable expectation.

With a great deal less international splash than Barnard, Cooley was among those whose public profile soared in the early years of transplantation, but Cooley too had virtually abandoned the procedure by 1970.

In the late 1960s, two other exciting advances made waves in the world of heart surgery, and Cooley wanted part of both of them as well. In the early days, transplants made for high hopes and good press, but they were not the answer. DeBakey had never been a great fan of transplants, and his reticence was well-placed, believing from the start that the solution was an artificial heart: a totally artificial, manmade, mechanical pump. With his carefully nurtured government connections, DeBakey was able to secure significant funding to begin the research for this medical moonshot. The obstacles were great, but if they could be overcome, he could bypass the lack of donors and the ethical issues. And since the devices were made of non-reactive, inorganic materials, the lethal problem of rejection would be side stepped as well. That was on the table, but still in the formative stages.

But other exciting things were happening. The hot, new procedure was coronary artery bypass surgery. Attempts to revascularize blood starved heart muscle had long been a dream. Various laboratory schemes were reported for decades. Simply bypassing the blockages made the most sense. The first successful clinical case was reported in 1960, but was hardly noticed. Most attempts were quickly abandoned due to post-operative complications, particularly stroke. Finally, in 1967, René Favaloro, an Argentine surgeon working at the Cleveland Clinic, developed a method of bypassing the blockage in the coronary arteries with sections of the saphenous vein taken from the leg. It might have been just another operation and just another anecdotal report, but Favaloro had pictures.

Mason Sones, the imaginative radiologist at the Cleveland Clinic, developed cardiac angiograms, or X-ray movies that clearly showed narrowed arteries around the heart and the location of blockages. This allowed Favaloro to pinpoint the areas to be bypassed, and later provided proof of the restored blood flow around the blockage with post-operative angio-grams. Coronary artery bypass graft (CABG) was the first suc-cessful treatment for millions of Americans with severe coro-nary artery disease.

Once again, Cooley was quick to grasp the implications and master the technique. The Texas Heart Institute was inun-dated with enough work to fill the hospital beds and wait-ing lists. Bypass grafts quickly became the mainstay of cardiac surgery practices, and the patient pool grew exponentially. Patients flocked to the Texas Heart Institute. Beds were full, the schedule was full, and Cooley even hired the former chief of cardiology at Walter Reed to become the full-time medical director of the institute. The nearby Shamrock Hilton Hotel was dubbed "the Cooley Hilton" and chock full of his patients and their families. Cardiac surgery had gone from a media frenzy to a feeding frenzy.

Although Cooley made numerous contributions to the science of cardiac surgery, they were generally of a more prac-tical and immediate nature. Cooley was not a surgeon scien-tist in the Lillehei or Wangensteen mold. He was, in fact, the ultimate operating surgeon. He reaped the rewards of his good work, and he enjoyed them. There were no lean years. In 1958, just six years into practice, he and his wife Louise were able to buy a ranch about an hour from home. "Cool Acres," as it was called, was expanded and augmented over the years, and the Cooley family spent happy weekends there. Cooley, the dentist's son, in his cowboy boots and Stetson, had become a rancher. By 1960, Louise had had delivered their fifth daughter, and the Cooley's left Cherokee Street for a much larger home in the fashionable River Oaks section of Houston. A white, colonial affair, the house had a sweeping lawn and an entry framed by imposing columns.

Cooley made the most of his free time as well. The ranch weekends were a regular family getaway, and a beach cottage in Galveston was added. Cooley traveled to far-flung medical conferences where he was frequently the featured speaker. He enjoyed working, he enjoyed socializing, and life was good. At the Houston Country Club, Cooley played his share of golf and tennis, and he and Louise were welcomed by the Houston elite. He golfed with princes and presidents and delighted in the powerful and famous new friends he made. Among them were James A. Baker, III, a lawyer and power broker, secretary of the treasury, secretary of state, and white house chief of staff, whose first wife, Mary Stuart, Cooley had operated on for metastatic breast cancer. Baker referred to his friend as the "king of hearts." Cooley became friendly with President George H.W. Bush, with whom he golfed, and later, President George W. Bush. It was a time of rising national importance of Texas Republicans, and Cooley was in the middle of it. He was famous, sought after, and excelled at a profession he loved. Home life was satisfying, and their girls brought the Cooley's great joy, and occasional deep sorrow. The family functioned as a strong unit, that was rocked by the suicide of daughter Florence, in 1985, which dogged Cooley for the rest of a blindingly successful life.

Cooley's workday began at 7:00 a.m. He worked hard, and he worked long hours. But when his work was finished, often late at night, he was able to have a drink in his hand, turn off the stress, and enjoy life. He was easy to work with and easy to work for. He respected those around him, didn't raise his voice, and was always in total control at surgery. His self-confidence begat an attitude toward his associates and trainees that stood in sharp contrast to the abusive style of DeBakey. Both were perfectionists as surgeons, both were consumed by ambition and fed by oversized egos. But Cooley wore his ego with grace and humor, and it wasn't difficult to bear.

One longstanding joke from the Texas Heart Institute has an agitated assistant cornering Cooley, saying, "Dr. Cooley, Dr. Cooley, you have to do something. Serratia marcescens is killing our post-ops"

"Damn it, just fire the son-of-a-bitch."

Serratia marcescens is a bacterium and a rare cause of endocarditis, an infection of the inner lining of the heart. Though very likely apocryphal, the story speaks to Cooley's actual disinterest in anything other than operating. Despite his insistence on surgical laboratories at the Texas Heart Institute, they were for others. He was an operating surgeon, plain and simple.

When the plaintiff's attorney in a malpractice case, attempting to make a point of Cooley's arrogance, asked if he considered himself the best heart surgeon in the world, he simply replied, "Yes."

"Don't you think that's being rather immodest?" the attorney asked, trying to embarrass him in front of the jury.

"Perhaps" said Cooley, "but remember, I'm under oath."

The story, often repeated by Cooley himself, reveals his self-regard, as well as his sense of humor, and reflects an opinion largely shared by his peers. Cooley was quick to say that when a confident surgeon was asked to name the three best surgeons in the world, he should be hard-pressed to name the other two. Cooley might very well have been the best technical cardiac surgeon in the world. So subjective was the statement that only other cardiac surgeons were qualified to weigh in.

Lillehei believed that Cooley was innately able to simplify surgery, see what others didn't, and able to make heart surgery easier, faster, and safer. Few, if any, disagreed. To watch Cooley operate was to enjoy a ballet while others were square dancing. Another in-house joke at the Texas Heart Institute was:

"Who's the best surgeon in Texas?"

"Denton Cooley when he's sober."

"Who's the second-best surgeon in Texas?"

"Denton Cooley when he's drunk."

When patients are put on bypass, a plastic cannula, about half an inch in diameter is routinely passed into the aorta. The accepted method of introducing the cannula was to grasp the side of the aorta in a clamp, make a small hole in it with a scalpel, have assistants hold the hole open with retractors to allow insertion, and then unclamp the aorta. A traditional, safe approach which takes ten minutes to perform. Cooley held a scalpel in one hand, the cannula in the other, and simultaneously punched a small hole in the aorta and slipped the cannula into it. A five second procedure which required no clamping of the aorta, no retractors, and no assistants. No one else had imagined the ease of it.

With the Texas Heart Institute becoming a reality, the Cooley Hilton overflowing, and the operating schedule at capacity, the good times were rolling. The early years of congenital heart defect surgery meant saving desperately ill children, and it had been thrilling. The advances were monumental and lifesaving, but the patient population was too limited to sustain all the surgeons joining the field. DeBakey and Cooley were the leaders in aneurysm surgery, which kept them busy even after other centers had gotten up to speed. There were always patients seeking name brands, and DeBakey had seen to it that he was the name brand, with Cooley as his associate. But coronary bypass surgery meant thousands of needy patients surrounding every medical center in the country. Taken together, there was a full menu of surgical options that had become the practice of cardiovascular surgery.

The drama of heart transplantation had been the hot topic for two years, until the reality of rejection supervened. Cooley's two dozen cases were therapeutic challenges and publicity magnets, but few survived. DeBakey's statistics were slightly better, but few survived, and the future for irreparable hearts actually seemed to be the artificial heart. DeBakey had predicted so in 1965, before the dawn of the transplant era. He foresaw the difficulties of rejection, the limited donor pool, and the ever-present ethical storm clouds.

The artificial heart was another matter altogether. Who could find fault with replacing a failing heart with a mechanical device? Doctors wouldn't need to hover over moribund patients waiting for, or helping along, the moment of actual death. There would be no pleading with bereaved families for organ donation, and if the proper device could be created and mass-produced, it could provide all the hearts a heartsick country needed.

★   ★   ★   ★   ★

By the late 1960s, reality seemed to be gaining ground on the dream. Cooley, like many others, was intrigued by the idea. He was already extraordinarily busy, having added coronary bypass surgery to the menu of procedures he had mastered. He had become the go-to heart surgeon among those in the know, but he still lived in the public shadow of DeBakey. Cooley's office in the basement of St. Luke's was a stone's throw from DeBakey's at Methodist, but there was rarely any communication between them. That in no way implies that they were unaware of virtually every move made by the other. Baylor residents interacted with both, and senior staff constantly spoke among themselves. There were third person accounts of the comings and goings, and projects of each were freely discussed—just not between the estranged surgeons.

Increasingly, DeBakey felt the heat of his talented junior breathing down his neck for primacy. For his part, Cooley felt intentionally overlooked, unappreciated, and dismissively treated. Every request he made to the chief had been met with resistance or outright refusal. Things had gotten so heated at one point that when Cooley was denied what he believed a simple, and reasonable, request, he snapped at DeBakey, saying, "OK, have it your way Groucho," referring to DeBakey's nose, moustache, heavy eyeglasses, and striking resemblance to the comedian, Groucho Marx.

Face-to-face interaction was limited to departmental affairs, lectures, and official Baylor functions. Both men were full-time members of the Baylor staff, but they had been spending their operating days in separate hospitals within the Texas Medical Center since 1954. As Cooley's autonomous power base grew, estrangement and resentment escalated.

CHAPTER NINETEEN

THE ARTIFICIAL HEART

It wasn't at all surprising that Cooley hadn't been informed when DeBakey added the Argentine surgeon, Domingo Liotta, to his staff. The total artificial heart, or TAH, had been used in the animal laboratory at the Cleveland clinic as early as 1957. Liotta and his brother Salvador had been implanting their version of the TAH in the lab at the National University of Córdoba and their progress report at a meeting in Atlantic City stimulated a good deal of interest. DeBakey, who had been working on a related device, heard about the meeting, contacted Liotta, and secured a surgical fellowship for him at Baylor. From that point, there were several versions of events.

DeBakey had been working on a heart pump called the left ventricular assist device, or LVAD. This too was a wholly synthetic, man-made device.

As the name states, its function is to assist damaged left ventricles pump blood with greater efficiency and less stress. The idea was to take the burden of circulation off the left ventricle and allow the damaged heart muscle to heal.

Liotta thought he was coming to Houston to work with DeBakey on his artificial heart, which initially was the case. But DeBakey had secured new National Heart Institute grants for the development of the LVAD, not an artificial heart, and assigned Liotta to that project instead. Liotta felt he was the victim of a bait and switch and tried to make his case to the chief. DeBakey had lost interest and avoided talking to him about it. When the two finally had the long-avoided discussion, Liotta proudly brought along the new prototype he had developed in the lab. DeBakey dismissed Liotta and instructed him not to bother him with the subject again.

Disappointed and angry, Liotta visited Cooley to see if he could interest him in taking over mentorship of the project. Cooley grasped the many facets of the opportunity. He recognized the potential of the device as what was called a "bridge" to transplant, a tool for keeping the patient alive until a donor heart could be found. This was still the year of the transplant frenzy and Cooley had moved to its forefront. Liotta's vision was more long range than Cooley's. Although he recognized the value of the TAH as a bridging device, he had thought of it more as the beginning of a series of innovations leading to a permanent implantable device to replace transplants entirely.

In December of 1968, Liotta began working under Cooley with funds provided by Cooley's foundation, as well as what Cooley described as "a couple of small grants." The work proceeded in Liotta's lab at Baylor. Both Cooley and Liotta would later claim that they had taken pains to develop an entirely new device, separate from the TAH developed under DeBakey's NHI grant. Three months later, they had their new Dacron and Silastic device, and a new, air-driven, operating console to connect to the patient. The heart was tested on seven calves, one of which survived for forty-four hours. Calves cannot be sustained on bubble oxygenators for more than two hours. They simply die, with or without surgery. When Cooley employed his TAH, he became adept at the procedure and installed the device in an hour and a half, took the calf off bypass, and it lived. Confident that they were on the right track, another TAH was prepared for human use.

The opportunity to employ it was waiting among Cooley's hospitalized patients. Haskell Karp was a forty-seven-year-old cardiac disaster. A printing salesman, he had come from Illinois to Houston a month previously, seeking a surgical solution for multiple diseased valves, an enlarged heart rapidly failing from multiple heart attacks, and generalized atherosclerotic disease. Time was running out. The only hope Cooley could offer was a transplant, but a donor had not been readily available. With no heart available, and the patient dying, Cooley proposed a risky operation to Karp. He would try to excise a wedge of the diseased left ventricle and sew healthy muscle to healthy muscle in the hope of increasing pumping efficiency. Cooley harbored no illusions of the possibility of success and added that if the operation proved impossible, he wanted permission to insert an experimental device that might tide Haskell over until a heart could be found for transplant. The level of risk, physically and ethically, was obvious. So was the opportunity. Cooley had special consent forms drafted and signed by Haskell Karp and witnessed by his wife and a hospital administrator. Extensive conversations concerning the procedure and its risks were carried out in the presence of a prominent, local Rabbi until all eventualities had been covered. Cooley knew where this was going; it was not going to be a routine operation. After his experience with his first transplant, he prepared for the coming publicity wave, but he had not expected the tsunami that struck.

The surgery was scheduled for April 4. By that time, Haskell Karp's condition had deteriorated so drastically that he could barely breathe. Heart failure had overwhelmed his lungs and he was drowning in his own bodily fluids. Cooley was informed by his team that death was imminent. It was Good Friday, and he was at home with Louise and the girls when the call came. By the time he reached the operating room, the team was in place and waiting to begin.

Opening Karp's chest, Cooley remarked that he "had never seen a worse looking heart." After putting him on bypass, he cut out 35 percent of the diseased left ventricle and reconstituted the heart with heavy sutures, but a normal heart rhythm could not be restored. It was the point of no return. There were only two choices. Cooley elected to proceed with the installation of the TAH, rather than give up and let his patient die. By no stretch of the imagination could he not have expected that that would have been the case.

Cooley removed Haskell Karp's heart and proceeded to install the artificial heart. Sewing through Silastic—a vulcanized silicone rubber—was not the same as sewing human tissue; the sharp, curved cutting needles were not designed for the density and resistance, making the simplest moves a bit awkward. Cooley had done the procedure often enough in the lab that the technical difficulties were not a surprise. The feat was accomplished in a bit more than two hours, and it was early morning when the procedure was completed. Karp was disconnected from bypass, and the artificial heart took over. A normal heart rate and blood pressure were quickly achieved, and a man without a heart was awake and following commands.

The operation was a great success; Haskell Karp was alive and was the first human sustained by a totally artificial heart.

★   ★   ★   ★   ★

DeBakey read about the dramatic operation in the morning papers. He was in Washington for a meeting of the National Heart Institute and was blindsided and outraged by what had gone on in his absence. Phone calls to Baylor did nothing to calm him down. Neither Cooley, nor Liotta, had seen fit to inform him that they were working on a version of the TAH, and certainly not that they had planned to use it at the first opportunity.

★   ★   ★   ★   ★

The entire operation and the events leading up to it had been filmed for a documentary called *The Heartmakers*. Not surprisingly, Cooley held a press conference following the surgery. Juggling humility and pride, he tried to manage expectations. He first credited Liotta, and then made the point that Haskell Karp was tethered to the console that powered and regulated the "heart" which was meant to be a temporary measure, and that a wide search was necessary to find a suitable heart to transplant, for which he made a nation-wide plea. Shirley Karp, Haskell Karp's wife, made a similar and tearful plea, and the word was out. The media went wild. Possible donor hearts materialized, were evaluated, and found unfit. The hearts were too small or too damaged during transit for use. Lear jets had been dispensed to retrieve possible donors, and when the right match had been found, a series of aircraft malfunctions and change of planes had been necessary to finally deliver the donor to Houston with the heart in transplantable shape.

By the time the appropriate donor had been identified and brought to the operating room at St. Luke's, Karp had lived with the artificial heart for sixty-four hours. The transplant went well, but Karp, overwhelmed by the immunosuppressive medications, had developed pneumonia, complicated by renal failure. Haskell Karp died on April 8, 1969, thirty-two hours after the heart transplant he had waited for.

Cooley was hailed as a hero by a public spurred on by endless accolades in the press. He was the man of the moment, and he reveled in the attention. Innovators in the field, like Kantrowitz and Willem Kolff, who had been spearheading the TAH program at the Cleveland Clinic hailed the device and the surgery as a great step forward. Barnard praised Cooley's achievement as well. Shirley Karp joined the chorus and took every media opportunity to laud Cooley's efforts to save her husband. DeBakey was livid. Claiming that the operation was a publicity stunt performed with his device and without his permission, he began an unprecedented publicity blitz to discredit Cooley. DeBakey made his position known to surgical departments across the country, governing bodies of the American College of Surgeons, the National Heart Institute, and Baylor itself.

Cooley hid behind the shield he and Liotta had devised. He had funded Liotta's new device, DeBakey had abandoned his TAH project, no NHI money was used, and most pointedly, it was inserted as a lifesaving measure. In the end, Cooley was censured by the College of Surgeons and by Baylor, the latter for not requesting permission from the committee on research involving human beings. The censures amounted to little more than a slap on the wrist and did not affect Cooley's day-to-day practice. In fact, he had become more famous and more sought-after than he had been prior to the adventure.

DeBakey was relentless in his outrage, charging, among other things, unauthorized use of government property. He never commented on the medical necessity, claiming not to have firsthand knowledge. Cooley responded "...when someone throws you a life preserver you don't look at it to see if it's been approved by the government."

It was his position that a physician had the right, and in fact, the duty, to do whatever possible to save the life of his patient. In this case, he had tried resecting a portion of Haskell Karp's scarred, enlarged, inefficient heart, and when that failed, his choices were either let the patient die, or try to keep him alive long enough for transplantation. The only way to do that was by using the TAH as a bridge to transplant.

DeBakey was not mollified. Within weeks, he pushed through a requirement at Baylor that all clinical trials be approved by the Committee on Human Research. Not surprisingly, the committee was stacked with DeBakey appointees. Cooley reiterated that his job was to save lives, and a surgeon should be free to immediately implement extraordinary measures to attempt to save the lives of his patients. Using that stance and ignoring the accusation that he had intentionally set into motion a situation whereby the use of the LVAD was called for, he refused to sign the agreement, and severed all ties to Baylor.

Looking back on his actions, Cooley tried to defuse the situation. Several times in the months that followed, he attempted to discuss the incident with DeBakey. Each time, he was rebuffed by the chief, who refused to acknowledge his overtures. In DeBakey's world, Cooley had become a nonperson, and in due time gave up trying. But the sniping and accusations escalated. Within the Baylor–Methodist camp, Cooley's name could not be uttered in front of DeBakey without a tirade. In the Cooley household, the DeBakey name was simply not spoken. And so began the most spectacular feud in medical history.

It was a time that heart surgeons had become public glamor boys, in much the same way as the astronauts who preceded them, and the Silicon Valley stars who brought about the digital revolution. Everyone knew who they were. And the two giants of heart surgery, the two famous men who coexisted within the Texas Medical Center, training some of the same surgeons and inextricably joined in the minds of the profession and the public, did not utter a word to one another for almost forty years.

Through the ceaseless efforts of DeBakey and his sisters, who operated what amounted to a full-time publicity machine, the episode was neither put to rest nor allowed to die of inattention. Quite the opposite. The DeBakey team opened to public scrutiny what began as a private squabble at Baylor.

On April 10, 1970, a year after the Karp operation, the feud, which had been building a steady head of steam, erupted on the cover of *Life*. Most of the nation became aware of the warring surgeons and nearly everyone had an opinion. The press, which initially lauded Cooley, had gradually done an about face and saw his motives in a less favorable light. DeBakey, the surgeon scientist, garnered increasing public favor. The faces of the two surgeons on the cover of *Life* and the change in public opinion may well have helped turn Shirley Karp against Cooley, for whom she'd had nothing but the highest public and private praise.

Two years after the groundbreaking operation, the Karp family filed a $4.5 million malpractice suit against Denton Cooley and Domingo Liotta, claiming negligence, lack of informed consent, and improper experimentation. More than one year later, the case came to trial in Federal District Court. It was an uneasy year for Cooley, but he maintained his public posture. He was supported by Louise, well represented by the premier law firm in Houston, and had been kept very busy during the long wait.

The trial took place in June of 1972. The plaintiff's hopes rested on the testimony of Cooley's harshest critic, Michael DeBakey. However, DeBakey refused to testify. Instead of ordering him to do so, Judge John Singleton questioned him in chambers, where DeBakey claimed no personal knowledge of the case, no opinion of its appropriateness, and refused to conjecture. Based on the loss of what they had hoped would be their star witness, the Karp case against Cooley and Liotta was dismissed. A year later, the dismissal was upheld by an appellate court, following which, the United States Supreme Court refused to hear it.

DeBakey's refusal to testify, after having fanned the flames of professional censure, was seen as a line that physicians were loath to cross: testifying against one another in malpractice trials, particularly high profile, questionable cases. Perhaps DeBakey had been protecting his institution and his standing among other physicians rather than being protective of Cooley. Perhaps he was simply doing what he believed proper. Whatever the case, the animosity he harbored remained unabated for decades, and Cooley ceased his attempts at reproachment.

Another thirty acrimonious years passed before time began to soften their positions. Surgeons of great accomplishment

and renown now surrounded both men, and among themselves, they hatched a scheme for reconciliation. It wasn't easy
and it didn't happen quickly. In 2004, O.H. "Bud" Frazier, the
most important figure in Left Ventricular Assist Devices, organized a conference on the history of the LVADs at the Texas
Heart Institute, his home base. DeBakey had been an instrumental player in the development of the devices, and Frazier
invited him to speak. To the surprise of all concerned, DeBakey
showed up in hostile territory. He was ninety-three years old,
every bit his sharp self, and gave a very well-received talk. He
accepted the applause and congratulations, acknowledged
Cooley, and left without speaking to him. The enmity had softened, but it would be another three years before the two men
actually spoke.

CHAPTER TWENTY

ST. PAUL, JANUARY 15, 1973: THE TRIAL

Every seat in Judge Philip Neville's courtroom was filled for the federal tax fraud trial of C. Walton Lillehei. Reporters from as far away as New York City sat among the locals. The defendant was a celebrity in the Twin Cities and many in the courtroom owed their lives to him. From leaked details of the government case, it promised to be lurid entertainment.

Lillehei's fortunes had taken one bad turn after another. Mindless disregard for the business of surgery had begun an avalanche of misdeeds that brought him face-to-face with a felony charge for tax fraud that carried a maximum penalty of twenty-five years in federal prison.

From the moment he entered surgical practice in 1951, Lillehei paid little or no attention to the business side of his profession. Billing of private patients was not handled by the University of Minnesota, and each surgeon kept his own financial records. Lillehei's cash box was his desk drawer, and his bookkeeping records were index cards filed in shoe boxes. If he needed money, he cashed checks, otherwise they languished in the chaotic drawer. From the outset, finances had never been a problem, and as his fame grew, surgical fees rolled in more frequently. His fees were modest, and often went uncollected. His mind was always elsewhere.

Income tax issues, or issues from not filing or paying taxes, began in the early 1960s. When the IRS became aware of the irregularities, Lillehei began trying to catch up. In 1966, he filed and paid taxes for the years 1963 and 1964, but he never actually became current. The initial IRS investigator recognized negligence, and Lillehei promised to set things straight. By 1967, he was beginning his new chapter at Cornell and neglected to file for the previous two years. A new investigator was assigned to his case, and it was soon evident that the IRS was not going to look the other way. Examining those tax forms that had been filed, he found a pattern of personal expenses categorized as business gifts, including money to three girlfriends and a check to a Las Vegas prostitute that were written off as business. Family parties were miscategorized, and fees and honoraria were not recorded at all. The IRS calculated tax indebtedness as exceeding $125,000.

Lillehei was an easy target, and the IRS investigator did a wide-ranging and thorough job of exposing his transgressions. The United States Attorney, Robert Renner, took a hard line and was not above humiliating Lillehei to make points with the jury. Grateful patients reluctantly admitted having paid bills that Lillehei had marked as unpaid in his haphazard system. Testimony to the good he had done was sidelined. The Las Vegas prostitute swore that Lillehei's $100 check for secretarial services had been for other services entirely, and the courtroom erupted in laughter.

For the Minneapolis observers, this fall from grace was a tragedy in itself. For Kaye, it was the ultimate humiliation. She stayed away from the trial and distanced herself from social contacts as it progressed. Lillehei, dressed down for the trial, sat silently as he was dragged through the mud.

In defense of his client, Jerome Simon, Lillehei's lead lawyer, calculated that the use of Lillehei's name and the royalties from his inventions that had accrued to the University of Minnesota, which he had every right to deduct, more than covered his tax debt. In fact, Simon claimed, the IRS owed Lillehei more than $50,000 for the value of his unclaimed donations. Both of Simon's arguments had merit. The income the University received from sales of the DeWall-Lillehei oxygenator would have made the idea of taxes owed a moot point. But Lillehei, in assigning his royalties to the University, did not first register them as his property and then sign them over to the University, which was the letter of the law. So, despite obvious philanthropic intent, and with absolutely no attempt at personal gain, the claim was disallowed by the IRS.

A second issue involved royalties for the Kaster-Lillehei heart valve, for which Lillehei properly staked his claim before signing forthcoming royalties over to the University. The valve suffered a long gestation period, but by the time of the trial, more than $15 million in sales had been achieved. The company then producing the valve, despite its clear contractual responsibilities, had not yet paid any royalties to the University. The prosecutor harped on the fact that no royalties had been paid to the University, claiming that Lillehei was simply lying. In fact, the company had continued evading payment of royalties even as its president testified that Lillehei's stake exceeded $500,000, which would have totally changed the math of the case had it been paid on time. Years later, the company, Medical Inc., was ordered by the court to pay the University of Minnesota $3.4 million for the royalties gifted by Lillehei. It was a staggering sum that would have turned the federal case into a farce.

Near the close of the trial, Lillehei came up with surprise evidence. He had just recovered another shoebox of index cards which had been misplaced after the fire in his home. Simon set about making the most of the new evidence that showed significant numbers of unpaid bills, some of which had been at odds with testimony. The defense believed that despite the unnecessary character assassination, which could not be undone, and the blanket dismissal of millions in gifted royalties, they had turned the tide of the case.

During the following weekend, Renner enlisted two expert witnesses—one was a document examiner for the treasury department. Both testified that the charred index cards had been altered, and the numbers reflecting remaining balance had been changed. The surprised Simon tried to make light of these findings as nickel and dime issues.

Simon built the rest of his case on character witnesses, the genius and generosity of Lillehei, his obsession with saving lives, and his absent-minded professor behavior. Witnesses included the locally lionized Wangensteen, who testified that Lillehei had been responsible for saving thousands of lives, and these minor transgressions, if true, should be seen in light of the life of a great humanitarian. Lillehei saw himself as a victim in all but his unfaithfulness to Kaye. He never addressed the altered billing card issue, and inferred that the prosecution was vindictive over such minor offences at the behest of President

Richard Nixon, who had been angered by Lillehei's active campaigning for Hubert Humphrey in the 1968 election.

On Friday, February 16, 1973, after more than a day of deliberation, the jury in the US District court in St. Paul convicted C. Walton Lillehei of five counts of income tax evasion.

Prior to sentencing, Judge Neville had written to the Chief Federal Probation Officer about his concerns should Lillehei be convicted. He ascribed his erratic behavior to his peculiar personality, a succinct insight that those who worked with Lillehei had circled, but never quite stated so clearly. Among Neville's concerns was that medical organizations might savage him even though "his transgressions had nothing to do with his professional conduct."

This too, proved to be insightful.

Lillehei posted $25,000 bond and returned to New York, where his tenure at Cornell was winding down. He returned to Judge Neville's court room for sentencing on May 4. The Judge who had, prior to this case, publicly expressed his opinion that jail terms should be invoked on tax evaders, did just the opposite. He sentenced Lillehei to a fine of $10,000 for each of the five convictions, payable over five years, and six months devoting "...his full time, without compensation, to rendering charitable medical services in a hospital." Neville recognized both the factual weakness of the prosecution's case in considering the enormous value of Lillehei's gifts to the university, and the childlike manner in which Lillehei conducted his financial affairs, while making a very significant contribution to society.

Lillehei returned to New York to do his community service at the Brooklyn Veteran's Administration Hospital. Although another step down from his chairmanship at Cornell, the period proved oddly interesting to Lillehei. Located at Fort

Hamilton, the hospital sat on a parcel at the mouth of New York harbor, bathed in light, and facing the Statue of Liberty. It was a teaching hospital with several highly accomplished physician scientists at the tail end of their careers, and there were surgical laboratories. All of which might have provided some solace.

But Judge Neville's predictions regarding the scorn of the medical community had also proven correct. The State of Minnesota revoked Lillehei's license to practice for a period of five years, or until the conditions of his probation were completed, which they immediately announced to the local press. A similar motion in the State of New York, where Lillehei was practicing, suggested reprimand, but did not suspend or revoke his license to practice. Following the New York hearing, Lillehei's lawyers reopened the case in Minnesota, positing that the allegedly required suspension of license stated in the decision was not, in fact, required at all. The legal team was prepared to pursue the issue to court, and the board quietly reversed its decision without bothering to issue a formal declaration to the press, as they had done when suspending the license.

It was a significant victory, but merely one of many battles. An anti-Lillehei faction of the American College of Surgeons attempted to expel him from the august body. This was met with strong resistance led by Wangensteen, who prevailed. Prestigious cardiovascular societies whose membership had been tied so closely with Lillehei's pioneering work distanced themselves from him as well. Lillehei never fully understood or complained about being ostracized, just as he had not fully understood the politics of university life.

At the age of fifty-six, with his surgical career ended by irreparably compromised vision and relieved of his duties at the New York Hospital-Cornell Medical Center, Lillehei completed his community service in Brooklyn and returned to the Twin Cities a pariah.

The next two years of Lillehei's life were spent in social and professional exile. Even before Kaye endured the indignity of the trial, she had been aware of his infidelity and visited New York infrequently. She saw her task as maintaining their family in St. Paul. Even with a husband who regularly missed birthdays, holidays, and Thanksgiving, thoughtlessly brought colleagues home without warning for dinners and late-night drinks, she had been understanding and resilient. Lillehei's work was his calling and Kaye understood and respected it, but by the time Lillehei's life dissolved, Kaye had built a life of her own.

Unable to work as a surgeon, Lillehei was denied a teaching or research affiliation at the University. Despite entreaties from Wangensteen, Najarian wouldn't budge. He was a kidney transplant surgeon who cared little about what Lillehei had contributed. Najarian allowed what had been the mecca of cardiovascular surgery to wither shamefully away after Lillehei's departure. The number of cardiac cases performed by the department dropped from eight hundred annually to two hundred. Surgeons left and formed successful private groups, soon dominating the Minneapolis cardiac surgery scene. Having decimated the department, Najarian stood as the public face of cardiac surgery whenever successful heart transplants were performed, despite having nothing whatsoever to do with the operations. He restructured the department of surgery to concentrate power in his hands by means of the purse string. Every surgical fee earned passed through his hands, with increasingly healthier splits going to the department and channeled to Najarian's projects. It was a stinging blow to the Minnesota centric surgeons, and many of them left the department as well. Najarian, himself would later be indicted for federal crimes, but for the moment, he was in power and remained hostile to anything having to do with Lillehei. As usual, everyone was aware of this but Lillehei.

Politically inept as he had already proven to be, upon returning to the Twin Cities, Lillehei wrote to Najarian, pled for a meeting with him, and consistently misinterpreted lukewarm dismissals as hopeful signs. Just as he had been able to deal with having been ostracized in social settings without complaint, Lillehei's "peculiar" personality protected him from hurt that might well have been unendurable by most people. There was never talk of pulling up stakes, and the Lillehei's continued to dine regularly at the country club that Kaye liked so well, where her husband continued to be treated as a nonperson.

★　★　★　★　★

With no outlet for his surgical research, Lillehei spent his time keeping up with the literature and managing his investments. These, it turned out, were substantial, and growing. Despite having signed over the royalties on his pump-oxygenator and the heart valve, his personal investments were well-chosen and well-timed. He knew what he knew, and instinctively saw the next best thing. When Lillehei asked Earl Bakken, the hospital electrical tinkerer, to put together the portable pacemaker, Bakken's resources were strained beyond the income from his hospital work and his garage workshop. Lillehei loaned Bakken $20,000 for his new company, Medtronic. Based initially on the pacemaker, the company grew rapidly. The loan was converted to equity, which Lillehei sold for more than $1 million in 1974 dollars, the equivalent of $5.4 million in 2023.

In 1968, he invested in another pacemaker company, eventually called Cardiac Pacemaker Inc., (CPI). The startup was led by Manny Villafaña, who had worked as a salesman for Medtronic. The company's unique concept was adopting lithium batteries to power pacemakers. The switch from mercury to lithium power proved to be revolutionary. The short lifespan of mercury batteries required changing every three years. This meant more surgery and expense. Lithium batteries had a working life of up to ten years. It was a better idea, and Villafaña's company cornered the pacemaker market. Lillehei's $50,000 investment in the start-up brought him $2 million when the company was sold to the pharmaceutical giant, Eli Lilly, in 1975.

The Lillehei's were more than comfortable financially; they were wealthy. With no other outlet for his energies, Lillehei fielded numerous corporate opportunities. As Silicon Valley is synonymous with the digital world, Minneapolis was, at the time, the seat of medical device development. So much so that it had been nicknamed Minnesota Medical Alley, and Manny Villafaña was at the heart of it. After the Eli Lilly buyout made him a multimillionaire, Villafaña latched onto the third generation of a heart valve originally devised by Lillehei and improved upon by others. Villafaña bought the rights to the valve, started a company he called St. Jude to manufacture it, and hired Lillehei as medical director. Again, it was a propitious financial move. Lillehei made a major investment in the new company, and St. Jude became the world's preeminent manufacturer of mechanical heart valves. Every dollar invested in 1976 was worth $250 a decade later. Not only did Lillehei have a fascinating lifelong job, he became a multimillionaire many times over.

But Lillehei continued to seek an academic appointment. Although he could no longer operate, his mind remained fertile and unique. Numerous influential surgeons tried to intervene on his behalf, including Shumway, by this time the director of cardiovascular surgery at Stanford. Despite having known Najarian from California, Shumway's efforts were ignored. Wangensteen continued pleading the case until his own correspondence with Najarian became acrimonious.

Finally, a decade later, Lillehei was appointed clinical professor of surgery by Najarian. Why Najarian changed his mind at that time, or at all, was never revealed. But it would be hard to separate this change of heart from the public redemption Lillehei received from the academic, scientific, and medical business communities. That process of reentry into the world in which he had lived began dramatically in Boston, in April of 1979.

John Kirklin, the Mayo Clinic cardiac surgeon and Lillehei's friendly competitor from ninety miles down the road had been angered at Lillehei's treatment by men who could never qualify as his peers. At the April 13 meeting of the American Association for Thoracic Surgery, Kirklin took the podium to deliver his presidential address to an auditorium filled with every heart surgeon who could find his way to Boston, including Lillehei, whose presence surprised many of the attendees. Kirklin, who was not a play it by ear sort of individual, very likely knew Lillehei was in attendance, and may, in fact, have seen to it that he was. The topic of his presidential address was the beginning of open-heart surgery, which he had helped pioneer. Kirklin said the following:

Walt Lillehei with Dick Varco really began this modern era of cardiac surgery, with cardiopulmonary bypass, and I hope that he is present here at the meeting. He always was, and still is, a great hero of mine, because of his enormous ability and warm friendship. Dear colleagues, may I depart from my text to ask this great and pioneering cardiac surgeon to stand to your applause? Walt Lillehei, may we see you?

What slowly built into a thunderous standing ovation welcomed the stunned Lillehei back into the world he helped create. At sixty-nine years of age, diminished, with compromised vision, and not yet reinstated at his beloved University of Minnesota, Lillehei thus began his climb back to respectability. Imaginative bookkeeping and altered records would ultimately be forgotten. His trainees built surgical societies in his name, his value on the speaking circuit increased, and his personal fortune exceeded any reasonable dream.

Kaye Lillehei held the family together through the trying times. Her belief in Lillehei's special genius was unwavering. For his part, his personality did not change. He remained naïve to political nuance, convinced of his positions, and when he would speak of his trial, believed he had been convicted of "nickel and dime tomfoolery" in the face of having ceded the rights to a life's work and a veritable fortune to the University. His blind spots extended to his surgical record as well. He knew one direction: if something had to be done, it had to be done.

A decade later, the celebration of the resurrected Lillehei's eightieth birthday was attended by notables in the world of cardiac surgery. The speakers were led by Norman Shumway, who roasted the guest of honor to roars of laughter.

"Walt, you always remind me of Al Capone. You killed a lot of people, but they could only get you on tax evasion."

★　★　★　★　★

Publicly, Lillehei never complained. But when his star regained its glow, he was no longer one of the cardiac cowboys. More often, he was telling the stories to the young men who would bring cardiac surgery to the next level. Lillehei continued on as medical director of St. Jude, resumed his professorship, lectured extensively, and otherwise, lived a quiet family life in St. Paul.

The action in cardiac surgery had moved elsewhere.

CHAPTER TWENTY-ONE

PALO ALTO, 1966:
RADICAL PERSEVERANCE

The children seemed to be sleeping peacefully, but the discordant sounds of cardiac monitors confused the newly graduated nurse to tears. Alone on the overnight shift in the pediatrics unit, she had no idea where to turn or what to do, so she cried. Her panic was obvious to the tall man in rumpled scrubs, shapeless lab coat and tennis shoes, and he smiled as he ambled closer. The name Shumway on his name tag meant nothing to her, but she focused on the doctor part, and asked for help. Among the children in her care were four postoperative cardiac surgery patients, and their monitors made no more sense to her than an orchestra tuning up.

Shumway, checking on his surgical patients before going home, smiled, listened, and calmed the young nurse. Carrying a lawn chair in from the terrace, he made himself comfortable beside her, and began a tutorial on what it all meant, and how to deal. She learned, laughed, and forever remembered the night the famous Dr. Shumway had given up his evening to be her private tutor and psychologist.

Shumway held a unique place among heart surgeons. He was a genuinely nice man. He had a fierce wit, and the butt of his jokes was usually himself. He was doubtless the father of heart transplant surgery, though he always gave top billing to his various coworkers. His operating room was a very serious, very well-organized place, somehow described by everyone who worked with him as fun. His perseverance was legendary, and although Christiaan Barnard had stolen the brass ring from his grasp, he later laughed and said maybe it had been better that way; Barnard got busy doing other things and he got to keep working to make heart transplantation better.

★   ★   ★   ★   ★

The Shumway family business, The Home Dairy, in Jackson, Michigan, was a roadside diner up front, and an active dairy in the back. Born in 1923, Norman Edward Shumway, Jr. was an only child. A bright, "normal" small town boy educated in the local public schools, he was the star of an award-winning high school debate team and valedictorian of his class. But every spare moment was spent forty miles away, in Ann Arbor, working as a caddy and playing golf. Shumway began college at the University of Michigan two months before Pearl Harbor, initially planning a career in law. In 1943, after two years at college, he was called up from the army active reserves and shipped to an agricultural college in Texas, ostensibly to be trained as an engineer. The army required an aptitude test and, based on the results, he was given the choice of training as either a doctor or a dentist. Shumway chose the former, reasoning that it offered the greater likelihood of keeping him out of the dreaded infantry. He laughingly repeated over the years that "it was probably the first time an army aptitude test had been correct."

The army training led to three quick semesters of premed at Baylor University, in Waco, Texas, and then, circuitously, to Vanderbilt University School of Medicine as the war was ending. From Vanderbilt, Shumway arrived in Minneapolis in 1949, choosing to do his internship and residency in Minnesota, based on what he read about Owen Wangensteen. The odds of Shumway showering glory on the professor defied prediction. It was hardly a match made in heaven. And if the intellectual John Lewis irked Wangensteen with his comments, he was an amateur in the world of speaking his mind compared to his new, slightly younger colleague.

Wangensteen's program, heavy on research and light on clinical surgery as it was, prompted Shumway to say, "The hardest thing about cardiac surgery is getting to do it." But he signed on for his residency and PhD, and began working with the likes of Lillehei, Lewis, and Varco. As an intern on Lillehei's service, he had seen a hospital patient mistake Lillehei for the absent Wangensteen. Lillehei had gone about his business without correcting the mistake. When Wangensteen returned and made his rounds, the patient refused to accept that he was, in fact, the professor. Wangensteen left the bedside annoyed, whereupon Shumway, a lowly intern, draped his arm around the chief's shoulder and whispered, "You have to stop going around impersonating Dr. Wangensteen." Wangensteen didn't quite see the humor. Shumway loved the story, and it became part of his legend at Minnesota.

But it wasn't all fun and games. Shumway's residency was interrupted by two years of service in the Air Force during the

Korean War, which he owed the government for financing his medical education. His time in the Air Force was spent primarily at a base in Lake Charles Louisiana, the ancestral home of Michael DeBakey.

Returning to Minnesota with his wife and baby daughter, Shumway jumped onto the Wangensteen surgeon scientist treadmill. He did a year in physiology, a year and a half in the surgery lab, working primarily on selective hypothermia and cardiac rhythms, for which he earned his doctorate, and a mere two and a half years in clinical surgery, which qualified him as a cardiac surgeon.

Shumway, with his obvious intelligence and sense of fun, was a well-liked team member. In awe of the accomplishments of Lewis and Lillehei, he would often moan that "You have to invent an operation just to get on the surgery schedule." At the completion of his training, Shumway had a young family and he needed a job. The tradition at the University of Minnesota was to meet with the chief about placement in an appropriate position. If there were no faculty positions open at the university, Wangensteen arranged for his young surgeons to become directors of surgery at small, local hospitals, which he believed both elevated the local care and increased the reach of his program.

Shumway worked hard but was short on self-promotion. Though he spent nearly three years of his residency doing laboratory work, he wrote a meager seven papers during his training. In academia, one is judged largely by one's output of scientific papers. Evaluating his situation at their meeting Wangensteen asked of Shumway's meager surgical writings, "What about these seven papers?"

"Well, you could actually read them," Shumway responded.

Wangensteen then offered a position at a small hospital in St. Paul where there was no opportunity for laboratory work or open-heart surgery. Shumway passed.

Despite not having been one of the chief's favorites, Shumway loved his time at Minnesota. He had been a resident on Lillehei's service for the birth of cross-circulation, and even donated blood for Lillehei's cancer surgery—to which he credited every great success of Lillehei's career. He idolized John Lewis, whom he considered the best of the surgeons at Minnesota, and he had been witness to Lewis's rise and fall. He had been there to observe and work with the pioneers of open-heart surgery, including the pushy Christiaan Barnard, whom he held in low regard. And despite all, he had great respect for Wangensteen, whom he considered the most mediocre of surgeons, but the greatest of teachers and the most selfless booster of his young staff. Wangensteen referred to himself simply as the "Regimental water carrier"—making sure the troops had enough support.

In later years, Wangensteen always found his way into Shumway's talks. Although their personalities never clicked, Shumway considered Wangensteen the major influence of his career. That influence was again felt some years later when Wangensteen encouraged the Falk family to support Shumway's work and create the Falk Cardiovascular Research Center at Stanford. Ralph Falk was a practicing physician and a founder of Baxter Laboratories, the first commercial producer of intravenous fluids. The 52,000 square foot building that resulted from the generous gift would ultimately become the home of Shumway's labs and operating rooms.

★ ★ ★ ★ ★

After finishing his training, Shumway agreed to join the California practice of a thoracic surgeon he had met at a medical conference. Packing up their small apartment, Shumway, his wife, Mary Lou, and their three children headed west to the beautiful seaside community of Santa Barbara. Shumway knew little about the surgeon he would be working for, other than the opportunity to do cardiac surgery, plus the allure of year-round golf weather. The adventure lasted only six weeks. Shumway always begged ignorance as to whether he quit, was fired, or both, but it was a poor match, and he headed north to San Francisco looking for work.

Calling on friends and colleagues, he made the rounds of the major hospitals. An interview was arranged with Leon Goldman, chief of surgery at the University of California. A force in San Francisco, Goldman's professional prominence was later eclipsed by being the father of the future long-serving United States Senator, Dianne Feinstein.

The interview didn't go well.

"While I was telling him how great I was, he nodded off..."

It was 1958, and Shumway ultimately landed a $3,000 a year job operating the dialysis machines at night and working days in the surgical lab at what was then called the Stanford-Lane Hospital. The laboratory, a leaky roofed, poorly equipped affair, was a leftover, make-do setup pending the hospital's planned relocation to the main Stanford campus at Palo Alto. Shumway's intention was to develop a cardiac surgery practice, which proved to be slow in coming. Most of his work, other than operating the dialysis machines at night, was covering for vacationing surgeons and continuing his experiments on the effects of hypothermia on cardiac function, ventricular fibrillation, and heart viability. It wasn't at all what he had envisioned, but he managed to support his wife and children and was happy in California, even though his schizophrenic schedule left little time for golf.

His situation improved when Ann Purdy, a pediatric cardiologist married to the chief of surgery at Stanford-Lane became dissatisfied with the pediatric cardiac surgery at her husband's hospital, moved her practice to Children's Hospital, and invited Shumway to join her. At the start, she referred some of the less complicated congenital heart lesions to him. His first case was a straightforward ASD, which he performed under hypothermia, the technique he learned from Lewis. It had also become his field of interest in the lab. He was completely comfortable with the surgery and the technique of hypothermia and he became the cardiac surgeon of choice at Children's Hospital. But it was still a jury-rigged affair. For each case, Shumway and the residents packed a van and drove all their equipment from Stanford-Lane to Children's Hospital and back again. Shumway's surgical results were excellent, but the bulk of the adult cardiac surgery in the city was still controlled by Frank Gerbode, the esteemed, senior surgeon with whom Purdy had become disenchanted. In all, Shumway did fifteen open-heart cases at Children's Hospital and established himself as first-rate cardiac surgeon, not just a laboratory investigator.

In the lab, Shumway was joined by Richard Lower, a junior Stanford surgical resident who accompanied him on the trips to Children's Hospital as well. The outlook for the future became brighter still when the long-anticipated move to Palo Alto took place in 1959. The new medical center was designed by the famous architect, Edward Durell Stone, and brought Stanford's medical research, teaching, and clinical facilities under one, modern roof. It was a far cry from the San Francisco labs littered with buckets to catch rainwater.

Entrenched in San Francisco, Frank Gerbode refused to move his practice thirty miles south, and Shumway found himself the default director of the division of cardiac surgery within the department of surgery of the Stanford Hospital. As Shumway related the story, he was told the position would be his until a big name cardiac surgeon could be recruited. That never happened. Soon enough, Shumway would stand among the leading heart surgeons in the world. Splitting his work week between the operating room and the laboratory, Shumway excelled at both, and the search for a famous chief became just another amusing anecdote.

In 1965, Shumway was officially named chief of the cardiothoracic division of the department of surgery. By 1974, his standing had risen so powerfully that he was able to establish an independent department of cardiothoracic surgery at Stanford. He would remain chair of the new department until his retirement in 1993.

In his first few years at Stanford, Shumway's surgical results were equal to any, but he broke no new clinical ground. It was his laboratory work that had brought him to the attention of the scientific community. Having earned his doctorate studying the cardiac effects of hypothermia, he enlisted Lower to continue the work he had begun. In its most basic form, his plan was to cool animals beyond the Minnesota style traditional hypothermia, to stop the heart, clamp the great vessels, and learn. By 1959, they had been able to use hypothermia to extend the viability of anoxic dog hearts to an hour. Using the same techniques of selective cooling of the heart in the operating room, Shumway achieved excellent clinical results in more complex surgical procedures requiring extensive operative time.

The logical next step was not logical at all. The new hypothermia apparatus selectively cooled the heart by resting it in a cradle of cooling tubes. For want of anything to do while observing the lengthened viability of the cooled heart, Shumway and Lower decided to pass the time by removing, then re-suturing in place the unoxygenated, cooled, non-beating dog heart. To their surprise, the first dog survived, and more surprisingly, when its heart was restarted, it resumed beating in a normal rhythm. Shumway and lower had reimplanted a pulseless heart and had a living dog.

The laboratory ennui that often resulted from these experiments—waiting to see how long the cooled heart could tolerate a period of anoxia-would turn out to be the starting line in the race to heart transplantation.

The first surprising finding was that a heart could be cooled, removed, and replaced without damage. The second was that a heart removed from the body, and therefore with all connections to the nervous system severed, would spontaneously resume normal rhythm and normal physiological responses when reimplanted. No efforts had been made to restore nervous connections, had that even been possible.

The actual removal and reinstallation of the dog hearts had proven technically more difficult than expected due to the paucity of tissue for sewing the heart back into place. There was no anatomic leeway, eight separate anastomoses were necessary, and the suture lines bled furiously. The surgical needles used at the time were bulky affairs, wider at the base where sutures were loaded through a notch than they were at the cutting edge. The crude needles did damage to the great veins and left small, but significant defects that bled. Lower had the inspiration of using the heart of a second dog instead of replacing the original. Shumway devised a method for connecting the low-pressure atria of donor and recipient, reducing the number of connections necessary from eight to four, and leaving enough tissue for extra sutures where necessary to control bleeding. Post operatively, the dog was active, and the transplanted dog heart survived and functioned well for eight days before being rejected.

★ ★ ★ ★ ★

The new technique had not been a planned surgical experiment, just the result of brainstorming about dealing with the difficulty of sewing the heart back into place. It was 1959, and heart transplantation had not been the goal. The whole exercise began as a sidebar to stave off boredom while waiting to see how long the cooled heart could survive, but the implications could not be ignored. Connecting atrium to atrium made the operation significantly easier and would be the technique that Barnard would use eight years later and remain the gold standard for sixty years.

As a stand-alone surgical feat, the transplantation of animal hearts was done by Carrel in 1915, and Demikhov in the early 1950s. The big news was the improved technique and the use of immunosuppressive drugs to actually prolong life before rejection.

Shumway and Lower became aware of the clinical implications and began to alter their thinking. Early in the journey, the learning curve included documenting the survival time of cooled canine hearts from harvest to transplant. This provided crucial knowledge going forward toward human transplantation since the chance of donor and recipient being in adjoining hospital rooms was impossible to imagine on any scale. Experiments were devised to determine how long a harvested, cooled heart could survive without oxygen before the muscle would begin to breakdown.

To follow the progress of rejection after transplantation, Shumway devised a noninvasive method based on observing changes in the electrocardiogram. The Stanford team also devised a percutaneous method for myocardial (heart muscle) biopsies. These were performed through catheters inserted in the jugular vein that allowed them to accurately determine the state of immune response. What these bits of information did was give the transplant team enough knowledge of the state of rejection to alter the dosage of immunosuppressive drugs as necessary to control rejection. The dogs were living longer and longer as the protocol evolved.

In 1965, the year they published these findings, Lower moved to the Medical College of Virginia. Both Lower and Shumway continued working on relatively parallel courses, with Lower sharing the knowledge that Hume's Virginia team had accumulated to deal with kidney transplant rejection.

By 1967, Shumway had transplanted more than three hundred dog hearts, assembled a competent team, and expanded his knowledge of the rejection phenomenon and how best to control it. Transplanting the human heart was in sight.

On November 20, 1967, Shumway made his intentions known in the *Journal of The American Medical Association* (*JAMA*). "We think the way is clear for trial of human heart transplantation…we are more, or less, at the threshold of clinical application." He went on to state that the transplant would take place as soon as the appropriate donor and recipient could be identified. It was the first time so direct a statement had been published.

Not two weeks after Shumway's pronouncement, with little laboratory experience and nothing resembling a well-trained team, Christiaan Barnard took the concept, and Shumway's technique, to the operating room and performed the world's first human to human heart transplant.

The race was over.

Three days after Barnard's operation, Kantrowitz, at Maimonides Hospital in Brooklyn, also using Shumway's biatrial technique, transplanted the heart of an anencephalic infant into an eighteen–day–old boy under hypothermia. The child survived for six hours. Kantrowitz considered the operation a failure. But what defined a successful heart transplant? Was a human living for six hours sustained by the heart of another human enough to be considered a success? Was eighteen days the benchmark of success? Leaving the hospital? Resuming work? Living for twenty years? Surgical success was a technical exercise. Surviving the post-op period, a medical exercise, and managing rejection the looming issue. Until normal lifespan was achievable, success remained a moving target.

On January 6, 1968, a month after Barnard, Shumway performed what initially was called the first successful human to human adult heart transplant in the United States. His patient, fifty-four-year-old Mike Kasperzak, a retired steel worker, had been crippled with debilitating heart disease when he suffered a massive heart attack. The situation was desperate, and Kasperzak's cardiologist believed his only chance for survival was a heart transplant—the new phrase that had been on everyone's tongue for the last month. Kasperzak and his wife did not need to be convinced, and he grasped at his last lifeline.

Four hours later, Virginia-Mae White, a forty-three-year-old housewife, suffered an intracranial hemorrhage and was on life support at a hospital several miles away. Kasperzak was already hospitalized at Stanford. White, with her heart beating, was declared brain dead by outside neurologists and transferred to Stanford by ambulance accompanied by Edward Stinson, Shumway's chief resident. She was wheeled into operating room 12 on the second floor and prepared according to plan. Kasperzak was in room 13, across a short corridor. With donor and recipient in place, Virginia-Mae White was disconnected from the respirator that had been sustaining her. Stinson rapidly split her chest open and removed her beating heart. Holding the still warm heart in his hands, Stinson gently lowered it into a sterile bucket of cold saline, as was the Shumway technique, and carried it into the adjoining room. In room 13, Shumway had already removed Kasperzak's diseased heart, and he was being kept alive by a heart-lung machine. Staring into Kasperzak's splayed open heartless chest, and then at two pulseless human hearts in stainless steel buckets beside them, Stinson broke the silence.

"Do you think this is really legal?"

"I guess we'll see," Shumway responded, and proceeded with the three and a half hour surgery. He carefully sutured the atria, aorta, vena cava, and pulmonary artery to the corresponding anatomic stumps. With Kasperzak still kept alive on bypass, the cold, pale heart sitting in his chest was shocked. Nothing happened. Kasperzak's body, brain, and the muscle of his new heart were being perfused by the heart-lung machine.

They waited. Slow waves appeared on the EKG, but nothing happened. They waited some more. Finally, twenty-five anxious minutes after completion of the surgery, a strong pulse in normal sinus rhythm resumed.

Bypass was disconnected, the chest wound closed, and the normally unflappable Shumway was exuberant. He smiled, congratulated Stinson, stepped out of the operating room, and was surrounded by unexpected tumult.

Shumway had predicted things to come in a scientific paper, but he had made no announcement about the impending surgery and was truly unprepared for the media storm that met him. The secret was out before the operation had begun. As the transplant team was being hurriedly assembled, a member was called away from a wedding reception. This was long before the privacy of cell phones, and a reporter attending the function made the connection. What began as a snowflake of private information became an avalanche. From a window in the recovery room, Stinson saw reporters scaling hospital walls. Television trucks materialized from every corner, and the unprepared public relations department of the hospital scrambled to assign a media room to answer questions.

Fifty-three years later, Tom Brokaw, then a Los Angeles television newsman sent to cover the event for NBC remembered it well: "We were summoned on short notice to Stanford, and Shumway was this handsome, youthful professor with a lab coat and a cool, engaging style, as opposed to his South African competitor who got there first. It was all very Stanford-California casual, but with a cool overlay of genius."

The next morning, Shumway faced hundreds of reporters in a Stanford auditorium and was his usual humble self. "We have reached first base, so to speak, but our work is just beginning." If the public was unaware of how difficult it would be to complete the sports analogy and reach home, Shumway certainly was.

Ed Stinson took up residence beside Mike Kasperzak in the ICU. For the first few days, Kasperzak did remarkably well. He was able to communicate with his wife, first answering questions by facial expression, and then by writing notes. Shortly after the initial progress, it became a struggle just to keep him alive. Shumway was not surprised. Kasperzak had been in terrible health prior to surgery. The stress of the operation led to what can only be described as an all systems collapse, culminating in massive gastrointestinal hemorrhaging. Kasperzak died on the fifteenth post-operative day. It was unlikely that he had suffered an acute rejection reaction. In truth, Kasperzak had been too ill to be reasonably considered for transplantation, and a new heart would not reverse his overriding illnesses. The transplant was a last resort. Both patient and surgeon were willing to take the risks, and both knew that a successful, long-term outcome was highly unlikely.

After the immediate media uproar, Shumway found himself facing legal action from the Santa Clara County coroner, who threatened to charge him with murder for "killing" Virginia-Mae White, claiming that with her heart still beating, she was not legally dead. Exactly the reaction Shumway expected as he and Stinson looked across the two heartless bodies. In the end, the district attorney, the actual legal authority in the county, declined to press charges.

The issue of brain death versus absence of heartbeat remained front and center when a 1968 ad-hoc Harvard commission suggested that absence of brain activity met the definition of death. The commission's findings were generally accepted but did not become law in California until 1973. By then, it no longer mattered. Hospital ethics committees had already been operating under those assumptions with few challenges, but the point was virtually moot.

In the frenzy that began with Barnard in December of 1967, and through 1970, more than two hundred and seventy-four heart transplants were performed, with only thirty-four long-term survivors. Very few of those were measured in years. Of the one hundred forty-three transplants done in the first twenty months after Barnard's operation, only twenty-one lived more than six months. And for the most realistic look, of one hundred transplants done in 1968, fewer than half lived for more than nine days. The overwhelming majority of patients perished within the first year. Rejection and infection were usually the cause of death, although there were operative fatalities as well.

In December of 1970, three years after Barnard's operation, The American Heart Association called for a moratorium on heart transplantation.

Shumway, the most realistic of the transplant surgeons, driven by what he called "radical perseverance," refused to concede defeat. Virtually alone, Shumway and his Stanford team persevered through the 1970s, when most of the others had given up. They were leading the world in experimental work, as well as refining the procedure, the aftercare, and learning to cope with rejection. Stanford remained one of the few institutions continuing to receive NIH grants for cardiac transplant research. Shumway saw the future of heart transplants as a life-saving, life extending operation for the sickest, most hopeless heart patients. He continued to avoid the limelight and worked at making it work. As the father of heart transplantation who had spent a decade in the lab developing surgical techniques and anti-rejection protocols only to see someone steal his thunder, he wasn't about to walk away from something he believed could be bent to his will.

Initially, Shumway worked with the immunosuppressive agents at hand: prednisone, radiation, and 6-mercaptopurine. Each fraught with disastrous side effects and difficult to balance against the susceptibility to infection in the wake of effective doses. Monitoring his patients for evidence of acute rejection by electrocardiogram and myocardial biopsies, he learned to tweak combinations of the drugs against signs of rejection and titrate their dosages against the need for antibiotics. With careful post-operative care, he managed to prolong the lives of his transplant patients, continually testing better agents as they came along, but none were game changers. In the mid-1970s azathioprine, a new, more effective immunosuppressive agent, was added to the arsenal. It helped suppress rejection but had the dangerous side effect of suppressing the bone marrow as well, adding life-threatening complications to an already life-threatening situation. But the Shumway team continued to increase survival times with even the rudimentary tools available. It wasn't dramatic, it didn't make the cover of *Life* magazine, it didn't make Shumway a household name, but his patients were gradually living longer—until everything changed.

★　★　★　★　★

A fungus, tolypocladium inflatum, was the agent of change. The Swiss pharmaceutical giant, Sandoz, had an odd protocol for traveling employees. The company provided them with plastic bags, encouraging them to bring soil samples back from the places they visited. The objective was to study the soil for the presence of antifungal antibiotics with commercial potential. In 1970, samples from Wisconsin and Norway yielded related fungi that were found to have limited antifungal action, but surprisingly potent immunosuppressive activity. When laboratory testing proved encouraging, the active ingredient, called cyclosporine, was synthesized. Its mode of action was to moderate the activity of T-cell lymphocytes, the active cells in the immune response, and the backbone of the rejection reaction.

The next step after the laboratory was clinical trials in kidney transplantation. Encouraging early trials were marred by life-threatening side effects like lymphoma, but rejection was largely controlled. In 1980, Tom Starzl, one of the front line solid organ transplant surgeons, began trials using lower dosages of cyclosporine combined with steroids on a series of liver transplant patients. Eleven of his twelve patients lived for more than a year, which represented a dramatic improvement from the rapid, acute rejection deaths experienced previously.

The news traveled quickly through the small coterie of transplant surgeons. Excited by Starzl's report, Shumway began experimental use of the drug in heart transplant patients in 1980, also with surprisingly improved survival statistics. Based on the overwhelming clinical trial evidence, the FDA fast-tracked cyclosporine in 1983 and made it available for clinical use. By that time, Shumway was well on his way to modulating the effects of the high doses of cyclosporine being used. He followed the onset of rejection closely and juggled drug administration with increasing success.

In 1981, Shumway and Bruce Reitz performed the first successful heart-lung transplant, which kicked off the cyclosporine era. Their forty-five-year-old patient left the hospital and lived five productive years after her transplant. Twelve years earlier, Lillehei performed the same surgical feat at the New York Hospital, only to lose the patient to acute rejection a week after surgery. Cyclosporine had been the game changer.

By 1985, Shumway had an 83 percent one year survival rate for his transplant patients, and an even more impressive 70 percent three year survival rate. This was unimaginable only a few years previously. Cyclosporine and the great success at Stanford meant the end of the fifteen year moratorium in heart transplantation. The miracle of cyclosporine was not without complications, and deaths from lymphoma continued. With time and experience, the dosage of the drug was dramatically reduced, achieving greater efficacy with far fewer side effects. Heart transplants were back on the menu.

In the 1980s and 1990s, more than two thousand heart transplants were performed annually, which begat a new problem: the lack of suitable donors. There has never been a lack of patients at, or near, end-stage heart disease. If heart transplantation is to be the solution, it can only be so if there are hearts to transplant.

Shumway allegedly argued against the California motorcycle helmet initiative because it would deprive hospitals of much-needed organ donors. The sarcastic remark would have been harsh and insensitive, but not at all unlike the black humor shared by surgeons, at which Shumway excelled. Apocryphal or not, the comment does underline the desperate need for donor hearts and the anguish of those waiting at death's door.

With an enormous need and a dearth of donors, every available heart counted. In large measure, Shumway's contributions helped make it possible for many more hearts to be salvaged and viable. Each small improvement was the result of dedicated laboratory and clinical work. On the most practical level, the simple knowledge that a donor heart bathed in cold saline could survive several hours of travel time made it possible to find far-flung organs and jet them to immunologically compatible recipients. The familiar, almost comical image of a team in scrubs and lab coats rushing from a private plane lugging a Pelican picnic cooler with a human heart packed in ice was built on Shumway's work. Viability stretched to six hours and determined how far afield the search could go. Organ locating and genetic matching became the work of the Organ Procurement and Transplantation Network, which has made the process faster and more reliable. Criteria from blood type and HLA (Human Leukocyte Antigens, the six genes responsible for the immune system) to matching, to physical size of donor and recipient are considered by the database. The unfortunate reality was that although HLA typing was optimal, it was a complex procedure which took a week to perform, and there was never time to spare. In most cases, matching was limited to simple blood typing.

Shumway's matching techniques, protocol for monitoring rejection, his simplified surgical technique, and the use of selective hypothermia were adopted worldwide, and twenty-five years of "radical perseverance" made heart transplantation a life extending reality. The number of heart transplants done annually in the United States after rising year over year leveled off and then rose again to about 3,800 annually. The increased availability of donor hearts resulted from the tragedy of the opioid crisis. The new mean life expectancy of transplants exceeds ten years, and the procedure, now quite routine, is performed in virtually all major medical centers with a cardiac team. Heart transplantation remains the go-to treatment for end stage heart disease. And as thousands wait in vain for a matched donor, the development of a permanent mechanical device has yet to materialize. Cardiac surgeon Eric Rose, former surgeon in chief of Columbia Presbyterian Medical Center, who, in 1984, performed the first successful pediatric heart transplant, summed up the supply and demand problem perfectly: "Heart transplantation is epidemiologically trivial."

★　★　★　★　★

DeBakey, who saw the problems inherent in transplants from the very beginning, had predicted half a century ago that one hundred thousand people would have artificial hearts by 1985. But in the ensuing decades, Shumway and his vision carried the day. And just as DeBakey performed heart transplants, Shumway became interested in mechanical heart assist devices and artificial heart valves.

The contrast between Shumway, his contemporary cardiac adventurers, and the slightly senior DeBakey could not be more striking. Of the group, Shumway was by far the least self-centered and ego-driven. It was his nature to be self-effacing and eager to share the laurels with others. To hear him tell his story, one would think he just happened to be there. The proverbial man who took his work, but not himself, seriously, Shumway left behind generations of superbly trained cardiac surgeons spouting "Normisms" along the way. He was a man who was able to tell a resident, with a straight face, that "all bleeding eventually stops." The most repeated of the Normism, "a good surgeon can always find a way to get out of trouble. A great surgeon devises an operation that even an idiot can do."

Shumway's operating room was a happy place with a supremely confident, competent leader who felt no need to assert his importance by demeaning others. His responsibility yielding method of teaching was the polar opposite of both the abusive DeBakey and the insecure Barnard. He was neither a workaholic like Cooley, nor an unusual personality like Lillehei. His method of teaching put the heaviest imaginable burden on the residents. Traditionally, after the pioneering days of Lewis and Lillehei, cardiac surgery residents were fully trained general surgeons who then opted for two years of additional training as cardiothoracic surgery residents. In this manner, capable surgeons were once again at the bottom rung of the ladder, gaining responsibility as they progressed.

At Stanford, Shumway integrated his cardiothoracic program with general surgery. Good residents, like Ed Stinson, his resident on his first heart transplant, were doing heart transplants start to finish before ever performing a simple hernia repair. Total emersion and total responsibility for the patient was Shumway's rule. Often a rule that dominated every other aspect of their lives. At surgery, the first assistant stands opposite the surgeon, and knowing all the moves, makes the procedure go more smoothly for the surgeon. Shumway was proud to say he may not be the best surgeon, but he was the world's greatest first assistant. Responsible residents were given responsibility for surgery. Shumway stood as the competent but quiet first assistant, allowing the resident to perform the entire procedure as surgeon until a stumble or costly mistake loomed. He made every move as easy and natural as possible for the young surgeon, and in return, each trainee was expected to be totally knowledgeable and in command. No one wanted to lose the helm. For this, they worked as hard as they had ever worked in their lives, and perhaps ever would. At the completion of the procedure, the resident surgeon virtually lived with the patient, beginning with sleeping (or trying to sleep) in the ICU. It was a remarkable journey and a decidedly different way to grow surgeons.

William Brody, a Shumway trainee (and ultimately the President of Johns Hopkins) summed it up with:

> I never worked so hard in my life, and had so much responsibility at a young age. He was a brilliant teacher and a master psychologist. With his humor he always made it fun. To be in the operating room with Shumway was the height of your day...At a time when everybody made cardiac surgery seem complex, he made it seem easy.

Surgeons are meant to love their mentors. Every surgeon in every part of the world has indelible memories of their mentor, the person who trained them in surgery, the most dramatic of disciplines. In academic surgery, the goal was to produce talented, responsible surgeons who could serve their patients well and move the discipline forward. Beginning with the accomplished Richard Lower, Shumway trained seventy-six cardiovascular surgeons, including Bill Frist, who abandoned surgery and ultimately became Republican Majority Leader of the Senate. Twenty-two of his residents became chiefs of cardiovascular surgery at major institutions, a testament to his devotion as a teacher. He served them all well as a man of dogged science, superb surgery, and a model of hard work, responsibility, and humor. The rumpled presence in chinos and sneakers stood, in that way, and in perhaps every other way, in sharp contrast to the jet-setting man who beat him to the prize. That his eldest daughter, Sara, became professor of cardiothoracic surgery and led the heart transplant unit at the University of Minnesota, is its own editorial. That they collaborated on a well-regarded textbook, a great joy to him, is another editorial as well.

Although Shumway's 1951 marriage to Lou Stuurmans, a public health nurse, ended in divorce, he never remarried. The couple had three daughters and a son, each of whom became accomplished in their chosen fields. Shumway loved life in Palo Alto but was not oblivious to the industry growing up around it. Living at ground zero of the tech world, he made a point of warning his trainees against the seduction of industry. Proud as he was of his daughter, Lisa, an early principal of Sun Microsystems, he made a point of telling his residents he was training them to be heart surgeons, not entrepreneurs.

With a resume of more than 350 scientific papers, masterly teaching, and significant contributions to valve and aortic surgery, the father of heart transplantation structured his work in a manner suitable to his vision of a fruitful, happy lifestyle. Monday, Wednesday, and Friday were surgery days, Tuesdays and Thursdays research days. A schedule rigid in its own casual way. If a moment cleared, he could be found under a wide brimmed hat, carrying his bag around the Stanford golf course. He also golfed religiously in a Wednesday and Saturday foursome of hospital cronies. Along with Cooley and others, he belonged to the Senior Cardiovascular Surgical Society, a fancy name for the annual outing of golf-playing renowned heart surgeons. While Cooley golfed with presidents and secretaries of state, Shumway walked the Stanford course often enough to earn a plaque on the 12th hole. And he would generally rather talk about playing in the 1993 Pebble Beach Pro-Am than about transplants.

At his seventieth birthday party, Shumway said, "this is like being at a wake awake."

★ ★ ★ ★ ★

Norman E. Shumway died of metastatic lung cancer on the day after his eighty-third birthday. He was not a smoker. On the wall of his office hung the sign, "Where there is death, there is hope."

CHAPTER TWENTY-TWO

DEBAKEY

If Michael DeBakey was widely disliked, he was impossible to dismiss. The rise of Baylor College of Medicine and the Texas Medical Center were largely due to his influence and efforts. The continuous flow of government grants supporting all manner of cardiovascular research at Baylor were the direct result of DeBakey's influence in Washington, which began with four years in the army surgeon general's office, the creation of the Mobile Army Surgical Hospital (MASH), the leadership of the National Library of Medicine, and membership on numerous committees directing the national health, including his strong advocacy of Medicare.

For twenty-seven years, he worked eighteen-hour days, and six and a half day weeks. Between his 5:00 a.m. banana and café au lait, and the hamburger at his cluttered desk, DeBakey operated, visited patients, supervised laboratory work, wrote hundreds of papers, thought surgery, taught surgery, strode the halls, and walked the stairs, fingering and nibbling at the pocket full of pistachio nuts in his lab coat. He briefly discussed his day and the family with Diana as he ate a quick dinner before closing himself off in his study, drafting papers or preparing committee work.

There was no time for small talk, little time for family, and total dedication to his patients and his science. The love of mechanical things that gave rise to the DeBakey roller pump and various artificial heart devices carried over to fast cars. At various times, he roared the eight blocks from home to the hospital in a Ferrari 330 GTC Speciale, a yellow Lamborghini, a 350 HP Dodge Charger, and a Porsche—all gifts from grateful patients, and all of which he owned only until the expense of maintenance or boredom took over. A Rolls Royce Silver Cloud was among the gifts which DeBakey kept garaged after learning the cost of insurance on a $150,000 automobile. The Ferrari lasted two years, after which he sold it to his brother, Ernest, a surgeon in Alabama, who passed it on as well. An automobile worth something in the range of $5 million in today's market.

Despite his love for fast cars, he never wandered very far. DeBakey barely knew his way around Downtown Houston and put fewer than five thousand miles on the Ferrari. Most of his driving was to and from the airport. Trips to Washington were frequent and short, but still took him away from his patients, to whom he was devoted. There was only so much time and compassion a busy man could muster. His life was his work, and DeBakey made his choice early. Diana DeBakey made her choice as well. She understood, but sometimes understanding wasn't enough.

There were no nightly family dinners, no games of catch, and little fun for his sons to remember. Sometimes her husband's absentee parenting was infuriating enough for Diana to shout, "Maybe they should become patients, then you would care about them." But they persevered, and the marriage managed through the years under DeBakey rules. There was a greater mission, and everything else was secondary.

As shamelessly as he promoted himself and the Texas Medical Center, personal financial gain was never the goal. He raised money and earned money, but felt to his core that medicine was a calling not a business. Never a religious man, he identified himself an Episcopalian, but never attended church, believing that man's purpose was to leave the world better than he found it. The DeBakey's had always lived comfortably, and that seemed good enough.

His belief in medicine as a calling was also where his trouble began in Houston. Driving the private surgeons out of Baylor based on their academic mediocrity was a reality. But DeBakey also instituted a program where Baylor surgeons worked for the institution. Initially, he and Creech were the sole salaried faculty. Under DeBakey, all surgical billing went through Baylor and was split 50/50 with the surgeons, Baylor paying the cost of overhead. This didn't sit well with surgeons accustomed to minimal office expenses and free use of hospital surgical facilities, while retaining 100 percent of their fees.

When Cooley arrived, he too found the system unfair. With his speed and endurance, he quickly became the highest earner in the department and wanted to keep a bigger slice of the pie. The deal he forced on DeBakey and Baylor increased their percentages of fees earned. Through no effort of his own, DeBakey found himself earning more and was quite satisfied with the new arrangement.

Steadfastly disinterested in pursuing wealth, DeBakey made a few investments with his friends and family, which were always managed by others. In partnership with his brother, he bought one thousand barren acres two hours from Houston, which was operated as a cattle ranch overseen by one of his sons. With another son a drilling operation, started as a tax shelter, struck oil, and earned even more taxable income. He knew little of the details and had no intention of having it change his modest lifestyle. His responsibility to his four sons was met by paying for their education and sending them into the world. None followed him into medicine.

DeBakey dressed mostly in blue scrubs and a white lab coat bearing his embroidered initials, MED, which he hung outside the operating room on a peg beneath the same initials—also indicating the chief's reserved parking space. His scrubs and coat seemed ill fitting, and he often wandered the halls in his surgical cap with a mask dangling on his neck. He wore custom made, extra high heeled cowboy boots, gleaming white for the OR, black for dress. The extra high heels allowed him better visibility of the operative field, or at least, that was his rationale.

From a fashionable Italian tailor who'd been a patient, he purchased a single suit every year. In contrast to his overworked professor look in scrubs, the social DeBakey's dress was surprisingly impeccable. His suits and jackets fit perfectly, even his army uniform was precise and complimentary. DeBakey was aware of everything and every impression. It wasn't long before he shed the moustache and changed the heavy glasses for a sleeker look. As his receding hair turned grey, he colored it until old age. But scrubs and a lab coat were his identity. That was the way he was photographed and the impression he wanted to give.

With steady inflation, the growth of Houston's economy, and 1981 interest rates topping out at 21 percent, DeBakey's fees for each surgical procedure remained a surprisingly modest $2,500. He made exceptions for doctors, nurses, hospital employees, and their families, who were not charged. The well-placed and wealthy were asked to make generous donations to the DeBakey foundation instead of paying fees for services. The truly wealthy were cajoled into endowing chairs and contributing to building funds and research—a small price to pay for the gift of life. Others, like the Duke of Windsor, were notorious for never paying their bills, considering their custom the stamp of approval for all sorts of services and goods.

And despite being a non-believer, DeBakey treated clergy gratis, though he would frequently comment on the wealth lavished on the Vatican in the face of so much hunger and poverty in the world.

DeBakey was everywhere. His connection to the National Heart Act and the National Heart Institute beginning in 1948 brought him early to the attention of Paul Dudley White, the leading cardiologist of the day. A Harvard Professor who gained fame as President Dwight Eisenhower's cardiologist following his 1955 heart attack, White was the first to call DeBakey 'The Texas Tornado." The name stuck in the popular press, and the press stroked DeBakey's outsized ego.

In mid-twentieth century medicine, an unclear line existed between providing public information and actively seeking publicity. The latter considered grossly unethical behavior. DeBakey was the grand master of working both sides of the line: a physician of honest and loudly proclaimed ethics swathed in a holier-than-thou cape and wearing the underclothes of a shameless self-promoter. Whenever DeBakey moved cardiovascular surgery forward, not only were academic papers published in the best peer reviewed journals, but praising articles appeared in the lay press as well. DeBakey was instinctively front and center, even when events challenged his clear medical judgement. High tech cameras were installed in his new operating rooms, and press conferences were called before and after new procedures. His planned use of an LVAD in 1966 was preceded by press briefings in an atmosphere many likened to a media circus. He was a regular and comfortable television guest, and seemingly immune to criticism from other surgeons, local physicians, and even the *New York Times*.

During the rush to transplant, DeBakey was the man of sage counsel, applauding advances while holding back on entering the fray. In August of 1968, eight months after Christiaan Barnard's surgical coup, the Baylor team planned to perform a multiple organ transplant of heart, lung, and kidneys from a single donor into four different recipients. DeBakey learned what his team planned just before the start of surgery. His permission hadn't been asked, and he was wholly opposed. He confronted the team leader, Ted Diethrich, and ordered him not to proceed. Dietrich responded that Dr. Cooley was planning to do just such an operation, which stopped DeBakey mid-tirade. He reluctantly allowed the circus to begin but did not personally participate. At the press conference after the extraordinary procedure, DeBakey stood alone on the podium describing the operation and taking questions. Diethrich was never mentioned.

In 1968, Baylor College of Medicine left the parent institution of Baylor University, and DeBakey solidified his power by becoming successively CEO, president, chancellor, chancellor emeritus, and held the chair of surgery until 1993.

1968 was also the year that Debakey's two sisters, Selma and Lois, joined the faculty of Baylor. They were recruited from Tulane where they had distinguished themselves by teaching doctors how to communicate in the clear and cogent manner they called "the logic and language of medicine." The sisters also taught popular courses at meetings of the American College of Surgeons and were generally regarded as creators of a much-needed specialty. Both sisters became tenured professors at Baylor. With his sisters at his side, the publicity and the scientific communications escalated. DeBakey produced a torrent of medical papers and news releases over the next thirty years. In all, he published more than sixteen hundred scientific papers, books, and book chapters over the course of his long career.

The media was made aware of every newsworthy surgical or experimental advance, and often, the names of patients. Occasionally, interviews were provided prior to surgery, as in the case of the Duke of Windsor. But more often, patients grateful for the compassionate care, the time spent, the surgical excellence, and the simple fact that they were alive, became instruments of DeBakey's fame themselves. Some, like comedian Jerry Lewis, would become close personal friends. A chronic name dropper, his famous patients were frequently mentioned in talks and interviews, and he was not above discussing their cases in public. Joe Louis, King Leopold of Belgium, and Boris Yeltsin, President of Russia, were among scores of others.

In April of 1980, DeBakey took part in the final act of the medical mismanagement drama surrounding Mohammad Reza Pahlavi, the Shah of Iran. Recently deposed from power and unwelcome everywhere, the Shah was registered under a pseudonym at the New York Hospital and underwent numerous procedures, including gall bladder surgery for jaundice, which left him with symptomatic retained gallstones.

Ultimately diagnosed with large cell lymphoma, the Shah had a dangerously enlarged spleen and painfully enlarged, cancer filled lymph nodes. Requiring radiation therapy to shrink the malignancies, the Shah was secretly wheeled through the maze of tunnels under York Avenue connecting the New York Hospital with the Memorial-Sloan Kettering Cancer Center where he was treated.

In an ongoing battle for authority, numerous physicians, including the American internists, surgeons, and oncologists fled or were fired. The Shah was finally hospitalized in Egypt, and DeBakey was selected to remove his massively enlarged spleen. DeBakey was chosen to perform the surgery largely because he was the most renowned and respected surgeon in the world. Never mind the fact that his area of expertise was no longer general surgery. In theory, however, the operation is a simple one, requiring the tying off and resection of the pedicle of blood vessels serving the organ, and simply removing it. However, this was not a simple situation. The Shah's spleen was ten times normal size and riddled with cancer. Several reports indicated that DeBakey nicked the pancreas during the surgery, setting off another cascade of problems ending with the death of the Shah.

In the reconstruction of events following the surgery, DeBakey denied responsibility, and the actual facts were buried in a laundry list of acrimony. With his reputation untarnished, DeBakey returned to Houston.

Most of DeBakey's high profile surgeries were within his sphere of excellence and had far better outcomes. The list of celebrities within the DeBakey patient circle was uncommonly heavy with Hollywood notables. Others were just friends, and he was not blind to the fact that he was a trophy friend just as much as they were trophies to him. Some, like comedian Danny Kaye, whom he met at a New Year's Eve party at Mary Lasker's New York apartment in 1963, became close enough with DeBakey to suit up in scrubs and observe him at surgery.

Social mobility was a two way street. DeBakey, a man too busy for vacations, happily flew to New York at the invitation of someone important to his career. Having won the immensely important Lasker Award, he was named to the Lasker Award jury, and then to head it, significantly elevating his power in the scientific community and exposing him to a wider world of achievers.

The walls of his office were covered with effusively dedicated photos of recognizable faces. The actress and singer, Marlene Dietrich sent a photo of her famous legs, thanking him for saving them by bypassing a blocked artery. After caring for Frank Sinatra's dying father in 1965, the singer was so impressed with the care and humanity offered that he became a generous donor to the DeBakey foundation and frequently referred patients, often paying their bills. Over the years, the Sinatra relationship grew into a close friendship that would soon change DeBakey's life.

★   ★   ★   ★   ★

DeBakey's interests flowed with the tide of cardiovascular progress, but his imprint was greatest in the vascular aspect of the developing specialty. His name was often associated by the world with procedures that had been devised or pioneered by others. But, with his numerous and significant contributions, not the least of which his Dacron aortic graft, scientific writings, and publicity, DeBakey became synonymous with vascular surgery.

The birth of cardiac surgery in 1953 came at a time when DeBakey was already famous for treating the previously untreatable aneurysms of the aorta. His vascular service had been growing based on his early interest in atherosclerosis, the disease that blocked blood vessels, and his new techniques to bypass blockages and restore limb saving flow in peripheral arteries.

One in one hundred children are born with congenital heart defects, but those twenty thousand represent a tiny population compared to the number of adults needing immediate aortic surgery. The most well-heeled and well-connected sought out the master aortic surgeon and inventor of the Dacron bypass graft. DeBakey was busy. He also recognized that open-heart surgery was moving too quickly to ignore. He attended every meeting and congratulated the pioneers, but he was in no hurry to join them. The watch and wait reticence marked the beginning of his rift with Cooley and would leave him a few steps behind the rush of new techniques.

It would be several years before he too began performing open-heart surgery, finally authorizing the acquisition of a bypass machine at Baylor. Although he joined the transplant party, for the next four decades, his research interests focused on LVADs and artificial hearts. In 1965, the "Texas Tornado" captured the cover story of *Time*, and DeBakey was already talking up the artificial heart.

As early as 1966, he began using mechanical left ventricular assist devices (LVAD) to supplement the pumping action of damaged hearts in an attempt to relieve the pressure of pumping and allow them to heal. Each attempt was a DeBakey orchestrated media event, with press conferences before and after surgery, and the entire procedure photographed and filmed. But the first two patients died, and even DeBakey centric Methodists clamped down on the publicity. Within the cardiac surgery community, the DeBakey show was not well-received and sniping comments about his showmanship were common. Bowing to the pressure, in the breakthrough third case, DeBakey's name was not mentioned in the press when he and Domingo Liotta installed an LVAD in a desperately ill patient on heart-lung bypass. The LVAD relieved the burden of pumping and the patient's heart healed sufficiently for the device to be removed and allow her to resume a normal life. In the ultimate medical irony, the healthy woman died in an automobile accident.

Subsequent attempts were not as successful, but when circumstances were dire, the device had proven its worth. The LVAD was not quite the total artificial heart DeBakey was seeking, but his success seemed to make the leap surmountable. It was at this phase that he encouraged Liotta to expand the concept into the total artificial heart, setting the stage for what was to be the most publicized, longest-lasting feud in medical history.

With the artificial heart still in the experimental stage, and left ventricular assist devices hardly everyday tools, attention focused on work being done by René Favaloro and Mason Sones that made coronary artery bypass surgery a reality. Surgeons now had an effective tool to fight back against coronary artery disease, the villain in the half million cardiac deaths that plagued America every year. With virtually no family immune, this new application of open-heart surgery returned all manner of rich dividends for all concerned. Heart attacks were prevented, or treated, lives saved, and cardiac surgeons became all-stars and wealthy to boot. Through the 1970s and 1980s, every cardiovascular surgeon in the world filled their days performing and improving coronary artery bypass grafts. Michael DeBakey, surgeon, scientist, empire-builder, and medical politician, joined that number.

Coronary artery bypass grafts, known by the acronym CABG, pronounced "cabbage" is a delicate operation performed under magnification, but once learned, is not inherently difficult. The success rate of the operation was exceedingly high from the very beginning. But it is serious surgery, and there are enough tragic consequences dealing with patients in a tenuous dance with death that the procedure could not be taken lightly. It was routine, but a stressful routine.

The coronary arteries are fairly small, the largest, the left common coronary artery, measures approximately 4mm in diameter, less than a 5th of an inch; it's small, but not quite microscopic. When the blood flow through a coronary artery is almost completely blocked, symptoms such as fatigue or chest pain on exertion can result. Total blockage results in destruction of the oxygen sensitive muscle that comprises the substance of the heart and results in a heart attack.

As early as 1945, a number of techniques to revascularize the afflicted heart had been tried with varying levels of success. None fully solved the problem created by blockage of the coronary arteries, particularly the left anterior descending branch of the left common coronary artery, whose blockage was so destructive it was known among cardiologists as "the widow maker." If the idea of bypassing the blockage did not originate with DeBakey, his mantra "If it's blocked, bypass it," foretold the story.

The first success bypassing a blockage in a coronary artery was reported in 1962, by David Sabiston, who used the saphenous vein, easily harvested from inside the leg, as the graft. Although there was no X-ray evidence to prove patency, the patient was reported to have a pulse beyond the graft before suffering a stroke and dying. Two years later, DeBakey, in a dire operative situation, resorted to a vein bypass graft and successfully salvaged the patient. Both physical and angiographic evidence of restored blood flow exist, but surprisingly, especially for DeBakey, nine years passed until he finally reported it in the surgical literature.

Then came Favaloro and Sones in 1967. By 1970, their mortality rate was less than 5 percent. With that, the world of cardiac surgery changed, and coronary artery bypass grafting was universally adopted.

The procedure was refined as it became clear that vein grafts, which were simply expedient biological tubes, became blocked fairly regularly a few years after surgery. The use of arterial branches of the aorta to graft a functional artery beyond the blockage of the coronary artery became the rule. The internal mammary arteries, which were expendable functionally, largely replaced saphenous vein grafts as the vessel of choice, and longevity increased dramatically. Other technical improvements followed, but the CABG was alive and well, and so were millions of patients.

In Texas, CABG patients filled the "Cooley Hilton" and DeBakey's Methodist Hospital built an additional unit to handle the patient traffic. The furor over the "stolen" artificial heart faded from prominence as the two separate heart institutions within the same Texas Medical Center entered open competition to capture the market. Houston became the shopping center for heart surgery in the 1970s. By 1972, Cooley's group had already performed 1,900 coronary artery bypass procedures, with a 98 percent survival rate. In 1980 alone, Cooley and company performed 5,000 coronary bypass operations. Cooley himself performed ten, or more, of the procedures daily and often oversaw thirty. The surgical production line had been honed to a science, with senior residents and fellows preparing the patients, opening their chests for surgery, and hooking them up to the bypass pump in preparation for the senior members of the surgical associates of Texas to take over the actual bypass, then leaving closure of the chest to the juniors. Polypropylene synthetic sutures allowed faster, friction-free, continuous suture sewing, rather than the original silk, or polyethylene sutures, which required time consuming, individually tied sutures. The procedure on the matchstick sized arteries was performed wearing magnifying loupes eyeglasses with mini telescope lenses and was totally routinized.

The DeBakey team was doing enormous numbers of cases as well. With eight new operating rooms, four of which were dedicated to DeBakey himself, their in-hospital census also exceeded one hundred patients. Performing several cases a day prepared by his staff as well, DeBakey, though thoughtful and skilled, simply never possessed his rival's uncanny surgical genius. As if unaware of the gap between them, he never alluded to it, nor would a word be spoken in his presence about Cooley's accomplishments. "Dr. Cooley this, or Dr. Cooley that," could actually lead to permanent exile. DeBakey continued to deride his staff, embarrass them publicly, and even drive young surgeons out of Houston, or, worse still, into the Cooley

camp. DeBakey's partner, George Noon, a well-respected surgeon even in the earliest days, became known among colleagues as "Goddammit" for DeBakey's constant grumbling...
"Goddammit Noon."

Legendary outbursts included, "I don't need any of you
incompetents to do an aneurysm. Go stand in the corner and
I'll do it." And, "If your mother had known you would turn
out this stupid, she would have drowned you at birth." Or, most
often heard, "If I had three hands, I wouldn't need you at all."

Many were ordered to leave the operating room and some
were actually fired from the program for minor infractions. The
professor was known to hold a grudge as well. O. H. "Bud"
Frazier defected to the THI after having been a DeBakey
scholar at Baylor, and DeBakey didn't speak to him for ten
years. As Frazier rose to the forefront of those miniaturizing and
improving the LVAD, the two had many occasions to meet in
and beyond the Texas Medical Center. DeBakey ignored him.
Finally, after Frazier presented at a meeting, DeBakey sought
him out. Correcting what he believed was a minor error, he
scolded Frazier with one of his favorite rebukes, "inattention to
detail is the hallmark of mediocrity."

Frazier, like many others, believed there was simply no
upside to interacting with DeBakey. "He was vicious, he was
vicious," Frazier commented.

DeBakey dismissed his behavior as that of a perfectionist—
and everyone wanted their surgeon to be a perfectionist.

★   ★   ★   ★   ★

By the late 1960s, Baylor was the go-to place for the best of
the aspiring cardiac surgery residents to train, as well as for

fully-trained cardiovascular surgeons seeking to learn from the leaders. But the atmosphere was toxic. These were grown men, and quite naturally, many fled for more pleasant environments. Among staff and trainees, DeBakey was very much respected, but not at all liked. To his patients, he was attentive, caring, and godlike. To other cardiac surgeons, he was both a scientific innovator and an inveterate publicity seeker. To the medical and political establishment, he was an open-minded, insightful leader. And to the press, he represented what he worked so hard to have them believe: that he was the future of heart surgery. None of these simplistic views of DeBakey was entirely correct. And none were entirely wrong. He was, in fact, all of the above.

While he too was performing multiple coronary bypass operations daily, DeBakey's professional interests lay elsewhere. In truth, he had been late to the party, and was over fifty when he began doing open-heart surgery on any scale. He had made his name as the great vascular surgeon, was not part of the early open-heart revolution, and had never been fully invested in heart transplantation. His imagination, ambition, and political influence were consumed with the ventricular assist device and the artificial heart.

DeBakey's prominence as a national figure grew in the 1960s and 1970s. He chaired the Albert and Mary Lasker Foundation Jury, sat on numerous national committees, staunchly supported Medicare, and was an advisor to President Johnson. He traveled widely and visited Moscow often enough to debrief and befriend Richard Nixon, the president he had worked hard to defeat. Diligent years in the Surgeon General's office, the Veterans Administration, and the National Library of Medicine kept DeBakey central to national health care policies, and often took an open stance against the American Medical Association, which solidified his credibility within the Democratic White House and congress. He utilized that credibility well in 1964 when he convinced the National Heart Advisory Council to prioritize the development of an artificial heart, and Congress to Appropriate $500,000, (the equivalent of $4 million in 2023) to the project. And although he proclaimed that by 1985 one hundred thousand Americans would have artificial hearts, he had all but abandoned the project in favor of the LVAD.

The transformative early years of coronary artery surgery altered the nature and economics of open-heart surgery, but the sea change for Michael DeBakey in was his private life.

CHAPTER TWENTY-THREE

CHANGES

In the early 1970s, Diana Cooper DeBakey developed angina, or chest pain caused by insufficient blood supply to the heart. It was usually brought on by exertion, and in most cases, the root cause was coronary artery disease caused by atherosclerosis. In February of 1972, suffering severe chest pain, she was hospitalized for tests at Methodist when she suffered a heart attack. DeBakey was in the operating room when he was informed. He rushed to her bedside but was unable to marshal sufficient emergency intervention to save his wife of thirty-five years.

The unperturbable heart surgeon became despondent. His routine had been shaken, and his supportive wife had been lost to a disease in which he was the resident expert. It became obvious to all that he was drifting into depression. Despite four sons and a surgeon brother for support, DeBakey continued to withdraw. Sleep was never something he seemed to need, nor savor, and feeling lost and uncomfortable in his own home, he began sleeping on a cot in his hospital office where he also took his meals alone. The office, on the ninth floor of the hospital, had been his private domain for many years, and it was routine for him to send out for his hamburger and eat lunch alone while working at his desk. Since the "stolen" heart incident, the office door was always kept locked. The only key was his own, and for a period of more than two years, the office became all but unapproachable to others; it was a place to hide from his grief.

As his depression became increasingly palpable, the DeBakey sons enlisted Barry, the youngest among them, who had been managing the ranch, to move into his father's home. It was an uncomfortable situation. DeBakey disliked his daughter-in-law and, rather than deal with the problem himself, he asked his eldest son to disengage the interlopers. It was typical DeBakey. The unfiltered, insulting task master at work assiduously avoided confrontation in his personal life.

Over the next eighteen months, DeBakey gradually resumed his frenetic routine. The many hats he wore in Houston and Washington filled every waking moment, just as they had when Diana was alive. He had little time to feel sorry for himself, and soon moved back into the old house on Cherokee Street where he was cared for by his long-time housekeeper. Visits from his sons became less frequent as they saw their father's depression abate. He began travelling more than ever and spent more time with his new friends.

Coming back to life, he happily accepted an invitation from Frank Sinatra to attend an eightieth birthday party for the comedian, Jack Benny. Flying out to Palm Springs for the weekend, DeBakey was installed in one of the nine guest rooms at Sinatra's lavish estate. As was usually the case, there were famous men and beautiful women at Sinatra's parties. Among them a pretty German actress whom Sinatra had never met who came along with an uninvited actress acquaintance of the host who heard there was a party. Sinatra welcomed both women, and introduced the German actress, Katrin Fehlhaber, to his famous surgeon friend. Although the thirty-two-year-old actress was beyond her starlet years, she was strikingly beautiful, and confident in the world of men. From the moment of their introduction, Katrin focused her attention on the surgeon, thirty-five years her senior. DeBakey was smitten. By the end of the weekend, Katrin Fehlhaber had invited herself to Houston for a complete "check-up," and DeBakey was in love.

Katrin arrived in Houston and stayed. She moved into the Cherokee Street house and was immediately at odds with the DeBakey family. Making the four sons feel unwelcome, she asserted control of the household with the smiling consent of her lover. By this time, the word was out among family and friends. The general consensus was that Katrin was at the very least an opportunist, but DeBakey appeared happy. His sons held their tongues and hoped the episode would pass. When, just a few months later, he informed them of his intention to marry Katrin, they investigated her background. Unable to locate any family in or around Hamburg, which she called home, the facts of her career did little to change their view of the woman who seemed destined to be their new stepmother.

Katrin had achieved more notoriety than fame in the German film industry, based on several roles in the early days of soft-core pornography. Other than these sexploitation films, she had appeared in a single television film, and was otherwise largely unknown.

Deciding to marry at a castle outside Hamburg, DeBakey arranged for his four sons, his sisters, and a few friends to attend the ceremony. From the bride's side, only the actor, Curt Jürgens, whom she knew peripherally, and had been a patient of DeBakey's, represented her. No family or friends attended the wedding. That might have been something of an indication of things to come, but the bridegroom was ecstatic, the bride beautiful, loving, and happy, and all hoped for the best.

Returning to Houston, DeBakey resumed his routine at Baylor and Methodist, but was a changed man at home. Dinner was no longer a quick affair followed by a long night of study and writing. He dined with Katrin, socialized with her, and the couple spent all their evenings together. Living in Diana's Cherokee Street house was not a comfortable environment for Katrin, and with her husband's understanding, she enlisted a German architect to modernize the old place and make it her own. By the time they were finished renovating, the house became something of an eyesore in the sedate neighborhood; remodeled and decorated fully in white.

Not particularly concerned with family finances, DeBakey deputized his eldest son, Michael, to see that Katrin always had $10,000 in her checking account. Only when checks began to bounce did it become clear that she had never balanced a checkbook before. But, lesson learned, and the money still continued to flow out as soon as it appeared, or sooner. Conflicts arose quickly, and others were enlisted to deal with them. When the garaged Rolls-Royce Silver Cloud, gifted by a grateful Indonesian patient, came to her attention, she demanded it delivered for her use. DeBakey, unwilling to stand the insurance or maintenance of the expensive vehicle, instructed Michael to sell it immediately and give the funds to his foundation. To deflect Katrin's anger, he instructed Michael to buy a new Mercedes-Benz for her and explain that the Rolls did not belong to them.

With her show business career over and her famous husband always busy, Katrin convinced him to fund a business importing and selling elegant, handmade children's clothing from Spain. It didn't take long to realize that the Houston market was not ready for $500 children's dresses, and the venture lost $650,000.

Then the cattle ranch owned by DeBakey and his brother, Ernest, began to interest Katrin, and after two quick helicopter trips, she decided to renovate the cabin. The idea held no appeal for either sibling. Rather than buy out Ernest's share, DeBakey decided that selling the property was the easiest way to say no to Katrin without confrontation.

In 1977, two years after they married, Olga Katrina was born. A daughter was a new experience for the sixty-nine-year-old father of four boys whose youth he had barely experienced. The baby brought him great joy and softened the edges of the increasingly difficult behavior of his new wife.

On New Year's Eve of 1978, Katrin's eccentricities brought near tragedy. The *New York Times* reported that fireplace sparks ignited a rug and the Christmas tree in the home of the famous surgeon. Katrin, Olga Katrina, and a maid fled the house safely, but DeBakey, who returned to help the others, was hospitalized for smoke inhalation and superficial burns.

The family told a different story. Apparently, Katrin insisted on decorating the Christmas tree with lit candles, which were allowed to burn through the night. By New Year's Eve, the tree was quite dry, and after the family retired, a candle ignited the tree. By chance, son Barry DeBakey, visiting a friend across Cherokee Street from the house, saw the blaze, called the fire department, ran into the house, aroused the family, and helped lead them to safety.

Katrin became increasingly high-strung and unpredictable, and her instability took its toll on the romance. A psychiatric evaluation indicated bipolar disorder, for which she was medicated, but frequently abandoned treatment. As her behavior varied from honey sweet to venomous and back again, acquaintances and family began to distance themselves. DeBakey was painfully aware of his situation but refused to separate from his wife and risk the loss of the young daughter he loved. The wedge Katrin drove between her husband and his sons widened over the years and the extended family gathered infrequently.

After the first three years with Katrin, DeBakey reverted to his old work habits. He had just turned seventy, was operating his usual full schedule—leading the medical school, chairing government committees, traveling and lecturing extensively—and still in the prime of his career. The early morning routine continued, as did lunch at his desk. His diet was nothing like the menus in the *Living Heart* books he coauthored with cardiologist Antonio Gotto. Hamburgers, Tabasco sauce, Snickers bars, pistachio nuts, and gumbo sustained him. Kofta, the spicy, traditional, Lebanese meat balls, were his favorite food. His exercise routine consisted of rapidly walking the stairs between the second floor operating rooms and his ninth floor office, a routine finally abandoned in his mid-eighties when he was presented with a private key to commandeer the elevator.

By his late eighties, DeBakey was operating less frequently and spending more time working on LVADs, the unrealized artificial heart, and still making news.

In 1996, at eighty-eight years of age, the vibrant DeBakey was called to Moscow to consult in the care of President Boris Yeltsin. Yeltsin was a big man and a heavy drinker with long-standing, sluggish thyroid function. He was anemic from prior internal bleeding, had barely survived a heart attack, and was in dire need of coronary bypass surgery, which his Russian doctors did not believe he would survive. DeBakey's medical politics and publicity had again served him well. His relationship with Moscow had begun in the 1950s when he invited Soviet surgeons to lunch at a meeting in Mexico. The lunch resulted in the Russians visiting Houston on their way home where they watched DeBakey in action. That led to a return invitation, followed by more than twenty trips to Russia. On one of his visits, DeBakey performed a quintuple bypass on Mstislav Keldysh, a renown Soviet nuclear scientist and President of the Soviet Academy of Science. The Academy, in turn, elected him as a member the following year. DeBakey's reputation loomed large in Moscow medical circles, and among the soviet heart surgeons who visited Houston was the surgeon caring for Yeltsin. Although he was not to be the operating surgeon, DeBakey brought with him all the necessary equipment for any eventuality, including staff and his partner, George Noon.

Yeltsin was hesitant to undergo an operation that his doctors thought he was unlikely to survive. But the depth and intensity of DeBakey's workup, his exalted reputation in Russia, and his confidence in the outcome convinced Yeltsin to agree. The success that followed allowed Yeltsin to stand for reelection and change Russian history.

DeBakey, in typical fashion, held numerous news conferences and was painted as an international hero. The grateful Yeltsin added a foreword to the Russian edition of the DeBakey and Gotto book, *The New Living Heart*, calling him "a man with a gift for performing miracles." But the greatest miracle was yet to come.

DeBakey operated into his early nineties when he finally put down the scalpel. He continued practicing medicine, directing his research labs, flying around the world lecturing and gathering awards with the energy of a man decades his junior.

CHAPTER TWENTY-FOUR

LIFE CHANGES FOR DENTON COOLEY

Denton Cooley's career took off like a NASA rocket and continued to gain altitude for thirty-five years. After separating from DeBakey and Baylor following the incident of the purloined artificial heart, his already healthy balance sheet was in the stratosphere as well. In an era of generous insurance reimbursement for aortic surgery and cardiac surgery and overseeing thirty CABG procedures a day, he yielded rich dividends. Cooley became very wealthy indeed. The River Oaks home was expanded, Cool Acres grew, and the beach house was soon joined by the classic Galvez Hotel on Galveston Island. Cooley sunk money into revitalizing the hotel and rode the Houston real estate boom with Rolls-Royces in the garage.

Rich as he was, he remained amusingly, if not pathologically, cheap. The man with a $9 million income in the 1980s arrived at a meeting at the New York Hilton from his economy hotel and was promptly hit on the head by the quarter he tipped the cab driver. Rubbing his head, he looked at the cabbie who shouted, "Keep it. You need it more than I do."

In addition to modest hotels, he insisted on sharing rooms, passed the dinner bill to his juniors, and was rarely known to reach into his pocket. While Cooley himself referred to his frugality as the result of living through the great depression, others laughed at the intense, money driven tightwad side of the great surgeon.

Like the arc of a rocket, Cooley's financial life tumbled to earth with the stock market crash of 1987. When the price of oil plummeted, Houston real estate followed. With tens of millions already invested or pledged, he bet heavily on a large real estate project with a son-in-law. The banks quickly felt the pressure of the free fall, called in the mortgages and loans, and Cooley, with $100 million in debt, was forced to declare personal bankruptcy.

In the reorganization process, he lost the hotel, the beach house, investment properties, and other assets. Cool Acres had already been deeded to the children, and Texas law allowed him to keep the River Oaks home and his enormous personal income. The press had a field day and the humiliation stung.

With his surgical production line intact, Cooley was quickly able to buy back the beach house and the expensive cars. The amusing side of Cooley peeked through when he quipped that the good thing about going bankrupt at sixty-seven was that it kept you young.

★   ★   ★   ★   ★

Day after day, twelve long hours of multiple surgeries, and quick desk top lunches of soup and frozen yogurt were balanced by a fully rewarding family life. Early in their marriage, Denton and Louise Cooley began referring to one another as "Darl," their shorthand for darling. For the expanding Cooley clan, it became DarlWorld. Cooley purchased homes in River Oaks for their daughters, they all used Cool Acres, and the extended family remained close at hand. All but Louise, their ophthalmologist daughter, who left Houston for Los Angeles with her real estate developer husband whose heavily leveraged project tipped Cooley into Bankruptcy.

The mid–1980s, marred by the suicide of Florence in 1985, and the Bankruptcy in 1987, stood as tough times in an otherwise storied life. Cooley was still the busiest cardiac surgeon in the world and enjoying it. He led the Texas Heart Institute, and the Denton A. Cooley Cardiovascular Surgical Society, and accepted visiting professorships across the globe.

Still handsome and erect as he aged, Cooley habitually removed his glasses for photographs, and combed his thinning hair more carefully over his scalp. His uneven smile became a bit more obvious, his features sharper under paper thin skin, and he remained an immaculate, attractive gentleman.

Cooley operated full bore until quitting surgery at age eighty-seven. He continued to tend to his non-surgical work daily and allowed himself Friday afternoons for golf. He lost only five workdays after surgery for a compressed nerve attributed to a lifetime bent over the operating table. In his later years, he dealt with colon cancer, atrial fibrillation, ablation, a pacemaker, and pulmonary emboli, without complaint, and through his mid-nineties, he remained an active player in the world of cardiovascular surgery.

Through a long career, Cooley amassed more accolades than award, but those bestowed were significant. Ronald Regan presented him with the Presidential Medal of Freedom, and Bill Clinton awarded him the National Medal of Technology and Innovation, but closest to his heart of hearts was the NCAA Theodore Roosevelt Award for the collegiate athlete who achieved national professional recognition. In Cooley's words, "I finally got recognized for being a good 'jock' as well as a good 'doc.'"

CHAPTER TWENTY-FIVE

DEBAKEY AT NINETY-SEVEN

Michael DeBakey spent the last afternoon of 2005 in his library preparing a lecture when he was jolted by a sudden, intense pain between his shoulder blades. Running through the differential diagnosis, he ruled out a heart attack and realized he was suffering from a dissecting aneurysm, among the most painful of surgical emergencies. His wife, Katrin, returning home from an aborted trip and seeing him on the sofa, pale and uncomfortable, called his internist and a member of his surgical staff. Both doctors rushed to the house, agreed with the maestro's diagnosis, and advised immediate hospitalization. On the theory that he had stabilized, DeBakey refused. A CT scan performed four days later confirmed the diagnosis of a 5.2 cm aneurysm, a measurement of a scale that indicated the need for immediate surgery. Again, DeBakey refused hospitalization, and on January 6, delivered his lecture at the Academy of Medicine, Engineering and Science of Texas. For the next two weeks, his doctors were unable to convince DeBakey that hospitalization was crucial. He was the boss, and despite all evidence that he was failing, he made the decisions.

Finally, dehydrated, short of breath, and in crippling pain, DeBakey relented and was admitted to Methodist Hospital. The aneurysm in his chest had enlarged to 6.6 cm, and still, he refused surgery. When it enlarged to 7.5 cm on February 9, DeBakey was unresponsive. The crisis point had been reached. George Noon insisted on immediate surgery. Earlier, DeBakey had told others he did not want surgery, and the hospital administrators were afraid to overrule what they believed were his wishes. Noon persisted. The anesthesia department refused to put him to sleep, not wanting to be responsible for killing the great Dr. DeBakey. An anesthesiologist who had worked with DeBakey for years was enlisted from the Michael E. DeBakey Veterans Affairs Medical Center, where she currently worked. Noon insisted that DeBakey had told him to do what he had to do. While Noon prepared for surgery, an emergency meeting of the hospital ethics committee convened to deliberate whether to allow the surgery in the face of the patient's wishes, and their culpability. Precious time was being lost. Finally, Katrin DeBakey stormed into the meeting uninvited and demanded that the surgery proceed immediately.

In the operation that followed, DeBakey's entire thoracic aorta, including the major vessels supplying the brain and upper body, were removed and replaced by a synthetic tube of precisely the type DeBakey himself had invented half a century before. It was an operation he had pioneered, and it was performed by a man he had meticulously, and often abusively, trained to perform it expertly.

★ ★ ★ ★ ★

Seven hours later, with a Dacron graft replacing his torn aorta and its major branches, a feeding tube perforating his stomach for nutrition, a tracheostomy attached to a respirator to breathe for him, and a dialysis machine aiding his poorly functioning kidneys, DeBakey was brought to the recovery room alive.

As expected for a man of his age and debilitated condition, DeBakey's post-operative course was stormy. Three months after surgery, on May 16, he was discharged and returned home. After two weeks at home, his condition had so deteriorated that he was again dehydrated and delirious. Noon advised immediate hospitalization. Katrin objected, then relented, then, as soon as he was hospitalized, insisted on taking him home again. Noon conferred with DeBakey's sons, and a court order was obtained bypassing Katrin and giving Noon sole authority over medical decisions concerning DeBakey.

By summer, DeBakey was walking unaided, and by year's end speeding through the corridors of Methodist on a souped-up electrical scooter, seeing patients and issuing orders. It was a sight that made even the most beaten down staff smile with joy. The ninety-seven-year-old legend survived the surgery, the oldest person ever to do so, but the course of events before and after surgery had been a tale of weakness, fearfulness, hesitation, self-preservation, and ultimately, the strength of the human spirit.

★ ★ ★ ★ ★

On January 16, a year after his surgery and some days after impetuously having driven up to the DeBakey home, Cooley sent the following note:

Dear Mike,

Congratulations on your miraculous recovery from illness and surgery. As time passes, I have a growing desire to meet with you and express my gratitude for the influence you have had on my life and career. Especially, I am grateful for the opportunity you provided me more than fifty years ago to become established at Baylor and to be inspired by your work ethic and ambition. Those years remain in my memory. I appeared at your house about ten days ago for this purpose. Mrs. DeBakey graciously received me but said that you were sleeping. If you are willing to receive me, I am available at your convenience.

Yours truly,

Denton

CHAPTER TWENTY-SIX

RAPPROCHEMENT

O n October 17, 2007, DeBakey rolled down the aisle of the fifteenth meeting of the Denton A. Cooley Cardiovascular Surgical Society to a thunderous standing ovation. He gracefully accepted his honorary society membership and clasped the outstretched hand of a smiling Denton Cooley.

Cooley spoke first. "I hope this is not just a temporary truce or a cease fire, but a permanent treaty between us."

DeBakey responded, "I am glad to be here for two reasons. One is, I'm alive. And the other, of course, is to get this award. Denton, I'm really touched by it. I'm going to put it in my library."

A few months later, when DeBakey was awarded the Congressional Gold Medal by President George W. Bush among bipartisan congressional leaders, Cooley attended as DeBakey's personal guest.

Several days following the ceremony, DeBakey presented Cooley with a replica of the gold medal and the following note:

> Dear Denton,
>
> I am enclosing herewith a replica of the Congressional Gold Medal given to me last week. I would like to share it with you, since I think you deserve a part of this award. Our pioneering work in cardiovascular surgery was jointly done by us, and the "first" successful clinical cases that were reported helped to usher in the specialty of cardiovascular surgery. We can take pride in that observation.
>
> With kind regards,
>
> Mike

Michael Ellis DeBakey died two months before his one hundredth birthday. He is buried in Arlington National Cemetery.

Michael Ellis DeBakey: Born September 7, 1908. Died July 11, 2008.

Denton Arthur Cooley: Born August 22, 1920. Died November 18, 2016.

Norman Edward Shumway: Born February 9, 1923. Died February 10, 2006.

Christiaan Neethling Barnard: Born November 8, 2020. Died Sept. 2, 2001.

Clarence Walton Lillehei: Born October 23, 1918. Died July 5, 1999.

EPILOGUE

———◦◦———

The second half of the twentieth century saw heart surgery from conception to maturity. While the Cardiac Cowboys were the most visible players on this well-lit stage, the invaluable contributions of others have been minimalized, or unrecognized, simply for the sake of telling this tale. Not acknowledging the story of the Cardiac Cowboys and what they accomplished would be like landing a man on the moon and keeping it a secret.

Their life altering achievements speak to both character and kismet. Dedicated, inspired, and driven, all were not only smarter than most, but were in the right place at the right time. Prominence and success did not simply fall into their laps, they were, for want of a better description, unusual. But, as one of the last active participants in their world, as O.H. "Bud" Frazier so aptly put it, in the end, "they were just people, like the rest of us."

The passing of the cowboy generation marked the end of the beginning of the odyssey. Simpler procedures with more complex tools have brightened the landscape. Blocked coronary arteries have largely yielded to internal stents inserted by interventional cardiologists. New heart valves introduced through arteries, or veins spare the drama, and trauma, of major surgery as well. But as much as the process has changed, a great deal remains the same. Congenital heart deformities are corrected surgically in very much the Lillehei manner, and more than seven hundred thousand pacemakers are inserted annually. Coronary bypass surgery remains a necessary and lifesaving procedure, and aneurysm surgery, like the replacement of the aortic arch that salvaged the ninety-seven-year-old DeBakey, remain the dramatic province of cardiac surgeons. Several thousand left ventricular assist devices are inserted every year, often as a bridge to the more than 3,800 heart transplants performed annually. The mean life expectancy of transplants has reached 13.5 years, with many recipients living their full expected lifespan. And the great savior, the artificial heart, remains a dream.

CARDIAC COWBOYS TIMELINE

---•---

- 1931. Boston. Mass. General. John Gibbon watches patient die of pulmonary emboli and begins a twenty-year search to develop a heart-lung bypass machine with an initial goal of excluding heart from circulatory system to allow surgery, which evolved to the idea of allowing heart surgery.
- 1934. Tulane medical student Michael E. DeBakey devises a continuous blood pumping device to expedite transfusions without damaging red blood cells. The machine becomes an integral part of the heart-lung machine.
- 1935. Gibbon keeps cat alive for twenty-six minutes on his bypass machine.
- 1938. Boston. Robert Gross performs operation to close patent ductus arteriosis, which normally closes at birth. He is celebrated for the operation, which is actually performed on blood vessels and not the heart.
- 1942. C. Walton Lillehei finishes medical school and a surgical internship under Owen Wangensteen at the University of Minnesota and enlists in the Army. Serves as surgical hospital director in North Africa and Anzio commanding MASH (mobile army surgical hospitals). MASH

units devised by DeBakey to get surgical care closer to the front where it was most needed.

- 1942–1946 DeBakey, on leave from Tulane, serves as surgical consultant to Army Surgeon General's Office. Where he develops strong relationships with federal government, ultimately resulting in significant influence and government support for his work.
- 1943. Gibbon meets Thomas Watson, chairman of IBM, who provides financial and engineering support for the next generation of heart-lung machine.
- 1944. Baltimore. Johns Hopkins. Surgeon Alfred Blaylock, pediatric cardiologist Helen Taussig, and lab assistant Vivian Thomas develop a procedure to alleviate symptoms of Tetralogy of Fallot, a usually fatal combination of heart and great vessel abnormalities. The operation gives new life to these "Blue Babies," but is not actually surgery in the heart, rather joining vessels outside the heart. Thomas, who is black, and a master surgeon, gets no credit. Blaylock and Taussig become celebrities. Denton A. Cooley, an intern at Johns Hopkins assists on the operation and begins a fascination with vascular and heart surgery.
- 1944–1945. Military surgeon Dwight Harken removes shrapnel from inside the hearts of 134 soldiers. This is the first recorded and repeated surgical entering of the heart. All patients survive, proving the heart is not "off limits" as was believed for centuries.
- 1945. DeBakey receives Legion of Merit for developing MASH units. Lillehei earns Bronze Star and returns to the University of Minnesota to resume his surgical training.
- 1948. Heart disease accounts for more than 500,000 deaths annually in the US, more than the total American lives

lost in the world war. President Truman signs the National Heart Act to combat heart disease.

- 1948. DeBakey becomes chief of surgery at Baylor in Houston. Truman converts Naval Hospital to Veteran's Administration Hospital under DeBakey.
- 1949. Norman Shumway begins surgical residency under Wangensteen at Minnesota. Lillehei becomes chief resident.
- 1950. Wangensteen sees open heart surgery as the new frontier and begins assigning residents to study possibilities.
- 1950. Lillehei diagnosed with lymphosarcoma of the parotid gland and undergoes extensive, mutilating surgery. Outlook grim.
- 1950. After a trying four-month recovery period, Lillehei returns to work as a junior surgical staff member.
- 1950. Toronto. Wilfred Bigelow published studies showing how hypothermia reduces oxygen requirements of the brain and allows time for experimental open-heart surgery with heart stopped.
- 1951. Cooley joins DeBakey's staff at Baylor. On his first day, he excises an aortic aneurysm and begins the development of modern aortic surgery at Baylor.
- 1951. Philadelphia. Charles Bailey successfully frees a "frozen" mitral valve with finger dissection after first four patients died.
- 1951. Clarence Dennis, Minnesota, using a variation of Gibbon's machine attempts open heart surgical repair of congenital defects. Both patients die and use is suspended.
- 1952. Philadelphia. Gibbon brings his heart-lung machine to human operating room. Machine functions well but child dies due to misdiagnosis.

- 1952. Minnesota. Lillehei experiments with azygos blood flow to retain perfusion of brain.
- 1952. Bailey attempts to repair an Atrial Septal Defect using hypothermia but patient dies of air embolism.
- 1952. Minnesota. First successful open-heart repair of defect. F. John Lewis repairs atrial septal defect under hypothermia. For a year, Lewis is the only surgeon in the world doing open heart surgery. Lillehei recognizes the time limitations imposed by hypothermia and searches for method that will allow more time for more complicated procedures.
- 1953. Gibbon uses heart-lung machine successfully. Next two patients dies and he stops doing open heart surgery.
- 1953. Minnesota. Lillehei, Warden, and Cohen develop cross circulation technique to gain more operating time.
- 1954. Minnesota. Lewis attempts two ventricular septal defect repairs under hypothermia. Both children die.
- 1954. Minnesota. Lillehei operates on Gregory Glidden for VSD under cross circulation. Operation successful, but the child dies of pneumonia.
- 1954. Lillehei's next two VSD repairs under cross circulation are successful.
- 1954. Lillehei corrects the Tetralogy of Fallot with actual open-heart surgical repair, not simply joining vessels outside heart as Blaylock had done.
- 1954. Minnesota. Donor mother has cardiac arrest during cross circulation operation. Mother revived. Another brain damage. Several patients die, including four Tetralogy patients. Lillehei working on bypass machine to replace cross circulation.

- 1954. Houston. DeBakey devises Dacron aortic graft to replace cadaver grafts in aneurysm surgery. Houston becomes world center for aortic surgery.
- 1955. Minnesota. Lillehei uses dog lung to replace cross circulation. Decides it is inadequate and begins building a simple $15 pump oxygenator with Richard DeWall.
- 1955. Minnesota. Cooley visits Lillehei at University of Minnesota and Kirklin at Mayo Clinic, where he has been using an improved Mayo–Gibbon pump with good results. Lillehei, having shown Cooley his new oxygenator, elects to do his case under cross circulation. Cooley decides to get into the action.
- 1955. Lillehei becomes the first surgeon to use artificial patches to repair large Ventricular Septal defects.
- 1955. Lillehei, Varco, Cohen, and Warden win the Lasker award for Medical Research.
- 1955. Houston. Cooley replicates the Lillehei-DeWall oxygenator and performs nearly one hundred surgeries in his first year.
- 1955. Minnesota. Lillehei completes his one hundredth open heart surgery. Patient dies of heart block.
- 1957. Minnesota. Lillehei uses pacemaker designed by Earl Bakken to successfully treat heart block.
- 1960. Lillehei and Bakken introduce portable, wearable pacemaker, which starts a worldwide industry.
- 1958. San Francisco. Norman Shumway begins work at Stanford, soon moving to Palo Alto. Shumway and Richard Lower begin experimental heart transplants while doing other experiments.
- 1960. Minnesota. Lillehei completes his 1,000th open heart surgery.

- 1960. Artificial heart valves are developed by Albert Starr and Lowell Edwards.
- 1961. Houston. Cooley and Debakey split over recognition and money.
- 1962. Houston. Cooley begins Texas Heart Institute. His separation with DeBakey widens.
- 1962. Houston. DeBakey gets NIH funding for artificial heart program.
- 1963. Stanford, Cape Town, Richmond, and Brooklyn. Laboratory work on heart transplantation begins.
- 1965. Palo Alto. Shumway becomes chief of cardiothoracic surgery at Stanford.
- 1966. Minnesota. Wangensteen announces retirement.
- 1967. Minnesota. John Najarian becomes chief of surgery at University of Minnesota.
- 1967. Richmond, Virginia. Barnard visits Lower and Hume allegedly to learn kidney transplant anti-rejection protocol, but secretly plans heart transplant.
- 1967. Minnesota and New York. Lillehei leaves University of Minnesota and moves to New York City, where he is named professor and chief of surgery at the New York Hospital and chairman of the department of surgery at Cornell University College of Medicine.
- 1967 Cleveland. Sones and Favaloro at Cleveland Clinic use coronary angiography to identify and bypass blockages in coronary arteries, setting the stage for decades of life-saving coronary bypass surgery.
- 1967. Houston. Cooley does more bypass surgeries than anyone in the world.

- 1967. November. Palo Alto. Shumway announces that after 350 laboratory transplants his team is ready to perform the first human heart transplant.
- 1967. Cape Town, South Africa. On December 3, Christiaan Barnard shocks the world by doing the first successful human heart transplant. The patient, Louis Waskansky, lives for eighteen days. Barnard becomes a worldwide celebrity.
- 1968. Cape Town. On January 2, Barnard performs second successful heart transplant. Patient lives for eighteen months.
- 1968. January 6. Palo Alto. Shumway performs his first human heart transplant a month after Barnard.
- 1969. Heart transplants done around the world. Very short survival and all most die due to inability to control rejection and infection. Heart transplantation stopped at virtually all centers. Shumway and Lower persist.
- 1969. April 4. Houston. Cooley inserts a fully artificial heart into a human patient. The device is very similar to, if not exactly the same design as, the device developed by DeBakey and Domingo Liotta with federal research grants. DeBakey finds out when he is in Washington, DC, for meetings. Legal and moral battles ensue. DeBakey and Cooley do not speak for forty years.
- 1970. *Life Magazine* cover story of feud between DeBakey and Cooley.
- 1970. New York City. Lillehei removed as chairman at Cornell and chief of surgery at the New York Hospital. Remains a professor.
- 1970. Corornary bypass surgeries done at rate of more than 500,000 annually.
- 1973. January 15. St. Paul. Lillehei on trial for tax evasion and fraud. Faces possible twenty-five-year jail sentence.

- 1973. February 16. Lillehei convicted on tax evasion and fraud. Sentenced to $50,000 fine and six months of community service.
- 1973. New York. Lillehei performs final surgery due to failing eyesight. Lillehei is a pariah in the surgical discipline he pioneered.
- 1979. Kirklin recognizes Lillehei's contributions in his presidential address at the American Heart Association. Lillehei is once again recognized as the father of open-heart surgery.
- 1980. Palo Alto. Cyclosporine used for immunosuppression with great success. New dawn of heart transplantation with excellent long-term survival due to control of rejection.
- 1983. Cape Town. Barnard retires due to painful rheumatoid arthritis.
- 1999. July 5. St. Paul. Lillehei dies of prostate cancer.
- 2001. Barnard dies of asthma attack.
- 2006. Shumway dies of lung cancer, never having been a smoker.
- 2006. DeBakey undergoes surgery for dissecting descending aorta at age ninety-seven. He survives.
- 2007. Houston. Cooley retires after performing 100,000 heart operations.
- Debakey, ninety-nine, and Cooley, eighty-seven, make peace after forty years.
- 2016. Cooley dies at ninety-six.

ACKNOWLEDGMENTS

The passing of two generations have seen the incredible new world of open heart surgery become routine. Sadly, the story of its creation has unknown to the general public and often to the medical world as well. It is too important a part of medical history to drift into obscurity.

In the past a number of excellent books have covered various aspects of the subject drawing on information collected directly from sources present at the creation. I came to write this book some years later, while considering the story of the feud between doctors Cooley and DeBakey. I was soon struck by how much I didn't know, and felt an obligation to expand the scope of the project. The books I read initially formed the skeleton of the story I told herein. I owe a debt of gratitude to G. Wayne Miller for his excellent King of Hearts, The True Story of the Maverick Who Pioneered Open Heart Surgery: Daniel Goor, M.D. for The Genius of C. Walton Lillehei and the True Story of Open Heart Surgery: Denton A. Cooley, M.D. for 100,000 Hearts, A Surgeon's Memoir, Michael M. DeBakey for Memoirs, Remembering My Father, Michael E. DeBakey: Thomas Thompson for HEARTS, Of Surgeons and Transplants, Miracles and Disasters Along the Cardiac Frontier: and One Life, by Christiaan Barnard. The information overlaps, corroborates, and sometimes conflicts. I have sought a balance, leaning to the sources whenever feasible and in no time intentionally directly quoted, nor paraphrased, anything written without attribution. But the fact are the facts and no one owns the truth. None-the-less I apologize if I have slipped up and a few words sound like one or another of my predecessors.

My sources include archival recordings and filmed interviews with each of the "Cowboys." Many of these are available on YouTube should you be interested.

In addition to general published sources I scoured the medical literature and pestered friends for information. Although I had tangential acquaintanceships with three of the principals, I didn't really know them, so initially, I reached out to those who did. First among them was the legendary O. H. Frasier, M.D., "Bud" to everyone. In addition to having performed more heart transplants than anyone in the world, Bud is "mister left ventricular assist device." He is a great raconteur, generous with his time, and worked closely with Michael DeBakey early in his career, and with Denton Cooley for decades. What a source! This book opens with a single episode told to me by Bud which refers to a comment by Cooley to Frasier about the loss of human life so common in early open heart surgery. The actual comment was self-deprecating, black humor so common among surgeons. I have chosen to alter the setting and omit the juicy morsel lest you, the reader, get a stilted idea of what the loss of life meant to a pioneering cardiac surgeon. For that I apologize, but you get the drift.

In addition to Bud, front and center among the people to whom I reached out was my colleague and friend, Eric A. Rose, M.D. Eric, former Chief of the Cardiothoracic Surgical Service, and Professor of Surgery and Surgeon in Chief, and chairman of the department of surgery at Columbia Presbyterian medical center. Dr. Rose performed the first successful heart transplant in a pediatric patient, was at the forefront of immunosuppression, and remains a leader in the world of left ventricular assist devices. He also knew the players. With Eric the concept of a streaming video series grew. We partnered with the esteemed John Mankewicz and the Cardiac Cowboys podcast became a reality. From the podcast came interesting bits and pieces of the story from the numerous individuals we interviewed and recorded for the series. That effort was spearheaded, hosted, and written by the incredible Jamie Napoli and produced by Jamie, Joshua Paul Johnson, Jason Ross, Colin Moore, James A. Smith, Eric Rose, John Mankewicz, Dub Cornett and me. Interviews were organized by Jamie Napoli and usually included Eric Rose, John Mankewicz, and me.

The list of generous individuals who gave us their time and insight includes many who were intimately involved with the protagonists. They include, but are not limited to the following: Adam Barnard, Roberta Beach, Ceeya Patton Bolman, MSN, Dr. Morton "Chip" Bolman, Dr. William Cohn, Dr. Louise Cooley Davis, Michael M. DeBakey, Dr. Pamela K. Evans, Adrian Fischer, Dr. O.E."Bud" Frazier, Dr. Antonio M. Gotto Jr., Dr. Paul A. Laizzo, Dr. Gerald M. Lawrie, Dr. Craig Lillehei, Patric Liotta, G. Wayne Miller, Dr. James Moller, Dr. J. Philip Saul, Dr. Sara Shumway, Shirley Gidden Spinelli, Dr. Don Wukasch.

The mistakes in this volume are mine. I hope they are small ones and do not negatively impact the extra ordinary story of these individuals and their legacy.

Gerald Imber, M.D.
July 4, 2023